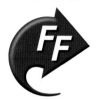

Fast Facts

✔ **KT-570-876**

BMA

Fast Facts: Pancreas and Biliary Tract Diseases

Second edition

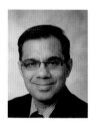

Manoop S Bhutani MD FASGE FACG FACP AGAF
Professor of Medicine, Walter B Wriston Distinguished
Professor for Pancreatic Cancer Research
Director of Endoscopic Research and Development
Department of Gastroenterology, Hepatology & Nutrition
The University of Texas MD Anderson Cancer Center
Houston, Texas, USA

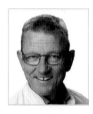

Peter Vilmann MD DSc HC FASGE
Professor of Endoscopy
GastroUnit, Division of Surgery
Copenhagen University Hospital Herlev
Copenhagen, Denmark

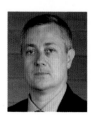

Adrian Săftoiu MD PhD MSc FASGE
Visiting Clinical Professor, GastroUnit
Copenhagen University Hospital, Herlev, Denmark
Professor of Diagnostic and Therapeutic Techniques
in Gastroenterology; Research Center of
Gastroenterology & Hepatology, Craiova, Romania

Declaration of Independence
This book is as balanced and as practical as we can make it.
Ideas for improvement are always welcome

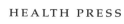

HEALTH PRESS

BRITISH MEDICAL ASSOCIATION

0825959

Fast Facts: Pancreas and Biliary Tract Diseases
First published 2006; Reprinted 2008, 2010
Second edition October 2017

Health Press Limited, Elizabeth House, Queen Street, Abingdon,
Oxford OX14 3LN, UK
Tel: +44 (0)1235 523233

Book orders can be placed by telephone or via the website.
For regional distributors or to order via the website, please go to:
fastfacts.com

For telephone orders, please call +44 (0)1752 202301.

Fast Facts is a trademark of Health Press Limited.

The publisher and the authors have made every effort to ensure the accuracy of this
book, but cannot accept responsibility for any errors or omissions.

For all drugs, please consult the product labeling approved in your country for
prescribing information.

A CIP record for this title is available from the British Library.

ISBN 978-1-908541-94-9

Bhutani S (Manoop)
Fast Facts: Pancreas and Biliary Tract Diseases/
Manoop S Bhutani, Peter Vilmann, Adrian Săftoiu

Medical illustrations by Dee McLean, London, UK,
and Annamaria Dutto, Withernsea, UK.
Typesetting by Thomas Bohm, User Design, Illustration and Typesetting, UK.
Printed in the UK with Xpedient Print.

List of abbreviations

AIDS: acquired immunodeficiency syndrome

AIP: autoimmune pancreatitis

ALT: alanine aminotransferase

APACHE: Acute Physiology and Chronic Health Evaluation

AST: aspartate aminotransferase

CA: cancer antigen

C5a: complement 5a

CBD: common bile duct

CCK: cholecystokinin

CEA: carcinoembryonic antigen

CFTR: cystic fibrosis transmembrane conductance regulator [gene]

CRP: C-reactive protein

CT: computed tomography

CTC: computed tomography cholangiography

ERCP: endoscopic retrograde cholangiopancreatography

ESWL: extracorporeal shock wave lithotripsy

EUS: endoscopic ultrasonography

FNA: fine needle aspiration

5-FU: 5-fluorouracil

GAP-43: growth-associated protein 43

GI: gastrointestinal

GRO: growth-related [protein]

HIDA: hepatobiliary iminodiacetic acid

ICAM: intercellular adhesion molecule

IL: interleukin

KW-PP: Kausch–Whipple partial pancreatoduodenectomy

MALT: mucosa-associated lymphoid tissue.

MEN-1: multiple endocrine neoplasia type 1

MIBG: meta-iodobenzylguanide

MODS: multi-organ dysfunction syndrome

MRA: magnetic resonance angiography

MRI: magnetic resonance imaging

MRCP: magnetic resonance cholangiopancreatography

NET: neuroendocrine tumor

NF-1: neurofibromatosis type 1

NSAID: non-steroidal anti-inflammatory drug

PAF: platelet-activating factor

PET: positron-emission tomography

pNET: pancreatic neuroendocrine tumor

PP: pancreatic polypeptide

PRSS1: protease serine 1 [gene]

PSC: primary sclerosing cholangitis

PSTI: pancreatic secretory trypsin inhibitor [gene]

PTC: percutaneous transhepatic cholangiography

SIRS: systemic inflammatory response syndrome

SPINK1: serine protease inhibitor, Kazal type 1 [gene]

TGF: tumor growth factor

TNFα: tumor necrosis factor α

TSC: tuberous sclerosis

US: ultrasonography

VHL: von Hippel–Lindau (syndrome)

VIP: vasoactive intestinal polypeptide

Introduction

Pancreaticobiliary diseases are extremely common, and all primary care practices will encounter patients with diseases of the various components of the pancreas and biliary tract. The symptoms of these diseases often see significant overlap with symptoms of other gastrointestinal diseases. Rapid differentiation, diagnosis, treatment and/or referral to a specialist must be made to avoid serious life-threatening consequences. It is therefore essential that every clinician has at least a basic understanding of the various diseases of the pancreas and biliary tract.

This book is an invaluable resource for primary care providers, physician assistants, nurse practitioners, medical students, medical residents, interns, house physicians and all other health professionals faced with the challenge of caring for patients with diseases of the pancreas and biliary tract. It provides a clear and concise guide to diagnosis and management. You will first gain an anatomic understanding of the systems involved, and will then be introduced to the evaluation of pancreaticobiliary diseases by means of history taking, clinical evaluation, and common laboratory tests and imaging modalities. Subsequent chapters rapidly build upon these principles, to equip you with the knowledge to recognize symptoms and signs, and select the appropriate laboratory tests and imaging modalities for accurate diagnosis.

Designed to help you correctly manage diseases of the pancreas and biliary tract and refer patients in a timely manner, since many will require referral to a specialist for medical or surgical intervention, this practical resource will also serve as an excellent grounding for further study of the specific topics discussed in each chapter. Since medicine is an ever-changing science, we advise readers to build upon their knowledge and stay up-to-date with the literature. The key references at the end of each chapter offer further and more detailed reading and, with this book, will provide a solid foundation for the field.

The pancreas

Anatomy. The pancreas is the shape of a small flat fish, 6–8 inches long and salmon pink in color. It lies behind the stomach, stretching between the duodenum on the right, to the center of the spleen (hilum) on the left (Figure 1.1). It is conventionally divided into the head, uncinate process, neck, body and tail.

Physiology. The pancreas is important for the production of:
- digestive enzymes – from the acinar cells
- bicarbonate – from the duct cells (to neutralize gastric acid)
- insulin – from the cells of the islets of Langerhans (essential for glucose control).

Epidemiology of pancreatic disease. In the year 2000 there were 1.15 million patients with non-malignant pancreatic disease in the USA.

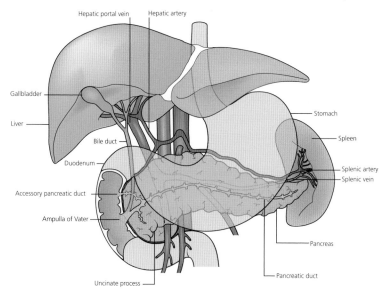

Figure 1.1 The anatomy of the pancreas and biliary tract.

Each year 125 000 North Americans present with acute pancreatitis, 100 000 present with chronic pancreatitis and at least 45 000 die from diseases of the pancreas. Pancreatic cancer is a highly lethal cancer and ranks fourth among cancer-related deaths in the USA. It is estimated that about 48 960 people will be diagnosed with pancreatic cancer and about 40 560 people will die of pancreatic cancer in 2015 in the USA.

In a study of a well-defined German population, the incidence rates for acute pancreatitis, chronic pancreatitis and pancreatic cancer per 100 000 inhabitants/year were found to be 19.7, 6.4 and 7.8 respectively. For acute pancreatitis, the highest incidence rates are in the USA and Finland. The incidence rate in Finland is 73.4 cases per 100 000 people. Similar incidence rates have been reported for Australia.

The biliary and pancreatic ducts

Anatomy. The main pancreatic duct joins the bile duct to form the common channel or ampulla of Vater (also known as the major papilla). In 90% of people, the embryonic dorsal and ventral pancreatic ducts are fused to form this pancreatic duct, meeting in the head of the pancreas. In the other 10%, the ducts drain separately into the duodenum (pancreas divisum) and the dorsal duct (known as the accessory duct) drains through the minor papilla. Small sphincters around the ends of the main bile and pancreatic ducts control the flow of bile and pancreatic juice, respectively; the sphincter of Oddi controls the outflow from the ampulla of Vater.

The gallbladder is tucked under the right liver lobe in the gallbladder fossa and is connected via the cystic duct to the common hepatic duct to form the common bile duct.

Physiology. Bile acids, essential for the absorption of fats and fat-soluble vitamins, are made in the liver and travel in canaliculi to reach the bile ducts. The intrahepatic bile ducts drain into the right and left hepatic ducts, which fuse to form the common hepatic duct.

Epidemiology of biliary tract disease. Gallstones are prevalent worldwide and are a considerable cause of morbidity and mortality.

They may cause acute biliary colic, acute cholecystitis or chronic cholecystitis, acute pancreatitis or cholangitis.

Gallbladder carcinoma is the fifth most common gastrointestinal (GI) cancer in the USA and the most common GI cancer in Native Americans. Incidence and mortality are very high in certain Latin American countries, especially Chile. Of the most commonly seen GI cancers in the USA, Europe and Australia, gallbladder cancer is the least common compared with other parts of the world. In most EU countries (with similar trends in the USA and Australia), mortality rates for gallbladder cancer have declined by approximately 30% among women and 10% among men, but mortality is still high in central and eastern Europe.

Bile duct cancer, or cholangiocarcinoma, may arise in the intra- or the extrahepatic biliary system, usually in people between 50 and 70 years of age. Sclerosing cholangitis affecting the biliary system may occur in association with diseases such as ulcerative colitis and in secondary form due to conditions such as AIDS. The gallbladder and the biliary system may also be affected by dyskinetic conditions such as sphincter of Oddi dysfunction and gallbladder dyskinesia.

Key points – anatomy, physiology and epidemiology

- The pancreas is 6–8 inches long and lies behind the stomach between the duodenum on the right and the center of the spleen on the left. It produces digestive enzymes, bicarbonate and insulin.
- The biliary system comprises the organs and ducts that store bile and release it into the duodenum.
- Pancreatic cancer is the fourth highest cause of cancer-related deaths in the USA.
- Gallstones are prevalent worldwide and a considerable cause of morbidity and mortality.

Signs and symptoms

The signs and symptoms of pancreaticobiliary diseases are usually non-specific. Patients typically present with variable symptoms related to the specific disease, ranging from chronic or intermittent abdominal pain (either biliary or pancreatic type), jaundice and/or pruritus due to obstruction of the biliary tract, nausea, vomiting, diarrhea or constipation, new-onset diabetes, fatigue, back pain and/or weight loss.

Biliary-type pain starts in the epigastrium/right hypochondrium, and is usually severe and penetrating with sudden onset and variable duration (15 minutes to several hours). It is sometimes referred to the right-shoulder area and associated with vomiting and/or nausea.

Pancreatic-type pain is felt in the upper abdomen, generally in the epigastrium, and radiates to the left and right, as well as the back. It is usually intense and steady.

Jaundice occurs when serum bilirubin levels increase to above 3 mg/dL. It may be gradual and associated with anorexia and weight loss. Jaundice can be easily observed at the level of skin and/or eyes (scleral icterus), and is sometimes associated with skin excoriation (due to pruritus).

Pruritus is the unpleasant sensation of itching associated with biliary obstruction.

Physical examination

The physical examination is complex and dependent on the suspected diagnosis. Patients with acute pancreatic or biliary pain (see above) tend to be anxious and cannot find a good comfortable position. An abdominal exam is important as it may reveal palpable masses in the right upper quadrant, or an enlarged gallbladder, due to obstruction by stones or a tumor.

Laboratory tests

Multiple tests with variable sensitivity and specificity are used for the differential diagnosis of pancreaticobiliary diseases. Usual laboratory tests include serum bilirubin, aminotransferases (transaminases), alkaline phosphatase, γ-glutamyltransferase, coagulation factors, amylase, lipase and, if pancreatic disease is suspected, blood glucose. These can highlight a possible cause for suspected biliary or pancreatic diseases.

Imaging

As the signs and symptoms of pancreaticobiliary diseases are non-specific, imaging is key to the diagnosis and management of patients. Imaging can clarify the presence and site of obstruction, as well as a possible cause in patients with cholestasis. Imaging modalities vary in diagnostic performance, technical success, complications and cost efficacy (Table 2.1).

Plain abdominal films (radiographs) have limited value, although they can show calcifications in the gallbladder or pancreas, as well as air in the liver or ileus. Oral cholecystography is relatively easy to perform, although its importance decreased with the advent of transabdominal ultrasound, which has a lower frequency of false-negative results.

Transabdominal ultrasound provides morphological information of the gallbladder, as well as the intra- and extrahepatic biliary tracts and pancreas. It is safe and cheap and can be performed at the bedside or emergency locations using versatile portable equipment. The accuracy for gallbladder diseases (especially for gallstones) reaches close to 100% but the technique is examiner dependent.

Transabdominal ultrasound is used in patients with obstructive jaundice to show the level of obstruction (dilated intra- and/or extrahepatic bile ducts) and the possible cause; nonetheless, the specificity is quite low for the differential diagnosis of stones in the common bile duct (CBD) compared with cholangiocarcinomas or pancreatic tumors larger than 2 cm.

TABLE 2.1

Imaging used in the evaluation of pancreaticobiliary diseases

	Recommended for diagnosis of:	Advantages	Disadvantages
Plain abdominal radiography	Rarely used but may demonstrate calcifications in gallbladder or pancreas	Widely available	X-ray exposure Not very sensitive for PB diseases
Transabdominal ultrasonography	Gallstones PB cancer Acute cholecystitis Acalculous cholecystitis Gallbladder polyps Gallbladder carcinoma Choledocholithiasis Caroli's disease Oriental cholangiohepatitis AIDS cholangiopathy	Widely available In expert hands it is sensitive for most PB diseases	Depends on operator experience Less sensitive in obese patients Cost effective
Endoscopic ultrasonography	Cholecystolithiasis (microlithiasis) CBD stones Chronic cholecystitis Gallbladder polyps Gallbladder carcinoma (staging) Chronic pancreatitis Pancreatic adenocarcinoma and other pancreatic focal masses Pancreatic cysts pNETs	Limited availability Very sensitive for most PB diseases The most sensitive method for limited disease (small tumors and microlithiasis)	Depends on operator experience Requires extensive training to obtain competence Very useful when combined with therapeutic ERCP in the same setting

(CONTINUED)

TABLE 2.1 (CONTINUED)

	Recommended for diagnosis of:	Advantages	Disadvantages
CT	Gallstones PB cancer Acalculous cholecystitis Gallbladder carcinoma (staging) Acute pancreatitis Chronic pancreatitis pNETs and pancreatic cysts	Gives a good overview of the PB region	X-ray exposure Small lesions may be missed
MRI	Gallstones Pancreatic adenocarcinoma pNETs and pancreatic cysts	Gives a good overview of the PB region similar to CT No radiation	Claustrophobia may prevent the examination Certain metal implants preclude MRI
Radionuclide scanning	Acute cholecystitis	Sensitive	Cost compared to transabdominal US Allergic reaction to dye
Dynamic HIDA scintigraphy	Chronic cholecystitis Acalculous cholecystitis	Sensitive	Cost compared to transabdominal US Allergic reaction to dye
MRI + MRCP	Gallbladder carcinoma (mapping) Pancreatic adenocarcinoma	Gives a good overview of the PB region No radiation	Claustrophobia may prevent the examination

(CONTINUED) 13

TABLE 2.1 (CONTINUED)

	Recommended for diagnosis of:	Advantages	Disadvantages
MRCP	Choledocholithiasis Biliary cysts Primary sclerosing cholangitis	Often first choice in patients suspected of choledocholithiasis No radiation	Claustrophobia may prevent the examination No therapy possible during the examination
ERCP	CBD stones Ampullary, bile duct and duodenal tumors Caroli's disease Pancreatic duct leakage, stones and strictures	Gold standard for many years At present only recommended for therapeutic use	Risk of acute pancreatitis, bleeding and retroperitoneal perforation

CBD, common bile duct; CT, computed tomography; ERCP, endoscopic retrograde cholangiopancreatography; HIDA, hepatobiliary iminodiacetic acid; MRCP, magnetic resonance cholangiopancreatography; PB, pancreaticobiliary; pNET, pancreatic neuroendocrine tumor; US ultrasound.

Although the pancreas is more difficult to examine due to its retroperitoneal position and frequent interposition of air or fat, various morphological features can be visualized, including calcifications, pancreatic duct dilation and the presence of pseudocysts or solid tumor masses.

Computed tomography and CT cholangiography can be used in patients with intra- or extrahepatic obstruction, although their accuracy in determining the cause of obstruction seems to be lower than for other imaging tests.

Multidetector helical CT and MRI are the methods of choice for the initial cross-sectional examination of the pancreas, including the evaluation of acute and chronic pancreatitis and early detection and staging of pancreatic tumors.

Multidetector helical CT is widely available and is often used initially in the evaluation of malignant pancreaticobiliary indications; however, for gallstone disease this method is less useful and magnetic resonance cholangiopancreatography (MRCP) or endoscopic ultrasonography (EUS) is preferred.

MRI is an exciting but expensive method that is useful for identification of pancreaticobiliary tumors. For some indications, such as evaluation of pancreatic cystic tumors, some clinicians prefer MRI because of its improved accuracy and detection of pancreatic cysts. MRI has the added advantage over CT of not exposing patients to ionizing radiation; however, due to claustrophobia, MRI is not possible in a number of patients and EUS has to be used instead. MRI can be supported with MRCP sequences that allow for high-accuracy examination of the bile ducts and pancreatic duct for diagnosis of stones and tumor masses.

MRCP has replaced endoscopic retrograde cholangiopancreatography (ERCP) as a diagnostic method and is also used as a screening method for the selection of patients that require therapeutic ERCP. Finally, magnetic resonance angiography has been proposed as a one-stop shop for the diagnosis, staging and resectability of pancreaticobiliary tumors, despite its relatively lower availability and higher costs.

Endoscopic ultrasonography is a high-resolution technique that combines endoscopy with ultrasound through the use of a high-frequency ultrasound transducer mounted at the tip of a specialized endoscope. EUS can detect CBD or gallbladder stones (microlithiasis) and therefore offers useful information in patients with suspected acute biliary pancreatitis or acute idiopathic pancreatitis. Detection of CBD stones using EUS is high (95%) compared with MRCP, thus avoiding invasive procedures and aiding the selection of patients for therapeutic ERCP. EUS has at least a similar accuracy with MRCP in the detection of CBD tumors and allows EUS-guided fine needle aspiration (EUS-FNA), which is followed by cytological or microhistological examination of the sampled material. Furthermore, EUS enables early diagnosis of chronic pancreatitis and the assessment of patients with advanced chronic pancreatitis by combining the evaluation of parenchymal and ductal criteria such as stones, duct dilation and/or the presence of pseudocysts. EUS has a higher sensitivity than other imaging modalities and facilitates the diagnosis of small pancreatic masses less than 2 cm. In addition, tissue diagnosis by EUS-FNA gives this type of imaging a distinct advantage over other cross-sectional methods. In experienced hands EUS is also used for therapeutic indications in pancreaticobiliary diseases. EUS can be used to either secure internal access and drainage of the bile ducts and pancreatic duct, or drain pancreatic pseudocysts and other fluid collections.

Endoscopic retrograde cholangiopancreatography combines endoscopy, for the identification and cannulation of the major papilla, with radiological examination after retrograde injection of iodine contrast agents at the level of the bile and pancreatic ducts. Although the complication rate associated with ERCP and the advantages of EUS and MRCP (see above) have almost completely removed the diagnostic role of ERCP, the method has retained its value in various minimally invasive interventional procedures such as sphincterotomy followed by stone extraction, lithotripsy and/or stent insertion.

Performing cholangioscopy and/or pancreatoscopy during ERCP has regained popularity in recent years because of the advances in image quality and endoscopes. These advances include the development of an ultra-thin endoscope that can pass through a duodenoscope and subsequently be introduced into the pancreaticobiliary duct system. Cholangioscopes are equipped with a working channel that allows biopsies to be taken for diagnostic purposes as well as therapeutic procedures such as stone lithotripsy and intraductal polyp snare resection. This makes both diagnosis and therapy of pancreaticobiliary diseases possible in one procedure. The method is used in selected patients with either retained stones or unclear stenoses suspected of malignancy.

Percutaneous transhepatic cholangiography involves puncture of the liver at the level of dilated intrahepatic bile ducts, followed by external or internal drainage of the bile ducts. Bile leaking and bleeding are complications seen in up to 10% of patients. This procedure is preferred in cases of failed ERCP or those with anatomic alterations that preclude papillary access by endoscopy. The method is now entirely used for therapeutic purposes since other less invasive and risky imaging modalities can be used for diagnostic purposes.

Key points – evaluation of pancreaticobiliary diseases

- The symptoms and signs of pancreaticobiliary diseases are usually non-specific.
- Imaging tests with varied diagnostic performance, technical success, complications and cost efficacy are used to confirm the presence, location and possible cause of pancreaticobiliary diseases.

Key references

Ashkar M, Gardner TB. Role of endoscopic ultrasound in pancreatic diseases: a systematic review. *Minerva Gastroenterol Dietol* 2014;60:227–45.

Chen J, Yang R, Lu Y et al. Diagnostic accuracy of endoscopic ultrasound guided fine-needle aspiration for solid pancreatic lesion: a systematic review. *J Cancer Res Clin Oncol* 2012;138:1433–41.

Giljaca V, Gurusamy KS, Takwoingi Y et al. Endoscopic ultrasound versus magnetic resonance cholangiopancreatography for common bile duct stones. *Cochrane Database Syst Rev* 2015;CD011549.

Miyakawa S, Ishihara S, Takada T et al. Flowcharts for the management of biliary tract and ampullary carcinomas. *J Hepatobiliary Pancreat Surg* 2008;15:7–14.

NICE. *Gallstone disease: diagnosis and management of cholelithiasis, cholecystitis and choledocholithiasis.* Nice Clinical Guideline No. 188. London: National Institute for Health and Care Excellence, 2014. www.ncbi.nlm.nih.gov/books/NBK258747, last accessed 17 August 2015.

NICE. *Suspected cancer: recognition and referral. NICE Guideline, No. 12.* London: National Institute for Health and Care Excellence, 2015. www.ncbi.nlm.nih.gov/books/NBK304993, last accessed 28 August 2015.

Rosenthal MH, Lee A, Jajoo K. Imaging and endoscopic approaches to pancreatic cancer. *Hematol Oncol Clin North Am* 2015;29:675–99.

Gallstones

Etiology and pathogenesis. Gallstones (cholelithiasis) are mainly composed of cholesterol, bilirubin and calcium salts. In Western populations the majority of gallstones are of the cholesterol type. These form when the cholesterol concentration in the bile exceeds the ability of bile to keep the cholesterol soluble by association with bile salts and phospholipids in the form of mixed micelles and vesicles (Figure 3.1). Non-cholesterol stones are pigmented black or brown and made up of calcium salts and bilirubin. Black-pigmented stones are more common in patients with cirrhosis or chronic hemolytic

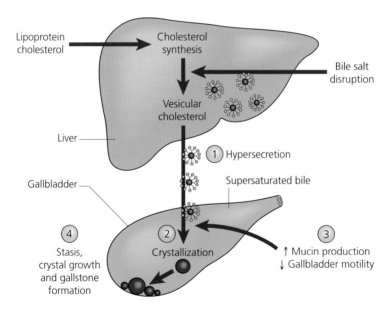

Figure 3.1 Pathogenesis of cholesterol gallstone disease: (1) over-secretion of biliary cholesterol by the liver in the form of unilamellar phosphatidylcholines vesicles; (2) incomplete micellar solubilization of vesicular cholesterol; (3) accelerated cholesterol crystal formation due to the presence of mucin and other still unknown pronucleating factors; (4) gallstone formation.

states, whereas brown-pigmented stones are more commonly primary bile duct stones found in association with infection.

Epidemiology and risk factors. Gallstones are a significant cause of morbidity and mortality worldwide. The prevalence of gallstones is greater in people over 40 years of age; women are at higher risk than men. In the USA, 5–8% of men and 13–26% of women have gallstones. Native Americans have the highest prevalence in North America, with more than 70% of Pima Indian women having gallstones; African-Americans have the lowest prevalence. European studies have reported the prevalence of gallstones to be about 10% in men and 20% in women, figures that increase to 30% and 40% respectively in older patients. Other risk factors for gallstones are given in Table 3.1.

Diagnosis

Symptoms and signs. Symptoms may arise from acute or chronic cholecystitis or choledocholithiasis (see Chapter 4), and some patients present with mild symptoms of intermittent right upper quadrant pain (biliary colic); these patients are at increased risk of gallstone-related complications. However, the majority of gallstones are asymptomatic and do not generally require treatment.

TABLE 3.1

Risk factors for gallstones

- Age > 40 years
- Female sex
- Estrogen replacement therapy
- Pregnancy
- Family history
- Obesity
- Diabetes mellitus
- Cirrhosis
- Crohn's disease
- Increased serum triglyceride levels
- Lack of exercise
- Drugs: octreotide, clofibrate, ceftriaxone
- Total parenteral nutrition
- Gastric bypass surgery

Laboratory tests are generally normal in patients with uncomplicated or asymptomatic gallstones.

Plain abdominal radiography is usually unhelpful, as 85–90% of gallstones are radiotransparent; however, it may reveal calcified gallstones in 10–15% of cases. Air in the biliary tree suggests an abnormal communication (fistula) between the gallbladder and bowel (usually the duodenum); air in the gallbladder wall (sometimes accompanied by an air–fluid level) indicates emphysematous acute cholecystitis (often in association with diabetes mellitus); and, rarely, a calcified ('porcelain') gallbladder indicates a premalignant condition.

Transabdominal ultrasonography is the preferred test for diagnosis of gallstones (Figure 3.2). Gallstones characteristically are highly echogenic with a typical posterior acoustic shadow (Figure 3.3). The sensitivity and specificity of transabdominal ultrasound are 98% and 95%, respectively.

Endoscopic ultrasonography (EUS) can detect even small gallstones missed by regular abdominal ultrasound. The method is often used instead of magnetic resonance cholangiopancreatography (MRCP) in the same setting as endoscopic retrograde cholangiopancreatography in patients with a high suspicion of common bile duct (CBD) stones.

Computed tomography. Although CT is not the preferred initial test for the diagnosis of gallstones, gallstones may be detected in approximately 30% of patients when a CT scan is performed for other reasons, such as abdominal pain or jaundice.

Magnetic resonance imaging has an accuracy of 90–95% in detecting gallstones, although this imaging test is usually not recommended for asymptomatic patients.

Surgical treatment of symptomatic gallstones and their major complications (acute or chronic cholecystitis, etc.) by cholecystectomy (removal of the gallbladder) is the definitive treatment for gallstone disease, usually by the laparoscopic route.

Laparoscopic cholecystectomy. This is a minimally invasive surgical procedure where the gallbladder is removed using a laparoscope. This is achieved through several small (one inch or less) incisions rather

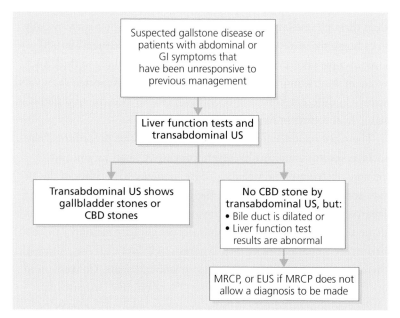

Figure 3.2 Diagnostic algorithm for symptomatic gallstone disease. The recommendations are dependent on the clinical situation, the symptoms of the patient and laboratory findings. CBD, common bile duct; EUS, endoscopic ultrasonography; GI, gastrointestinal; MRCP, magnetic resonance cholangiopancreatography; US, ultrasonography.

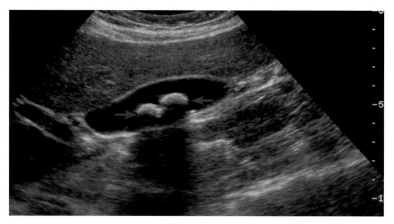

Figure 3.3 Transabdominal ultrasound of the gallbladder showing two stones with characteristic posterior acoustic shadow and surrounding sludge.

than through one large incision on the abdomen. The patient usually goes home the same day or the next morning. More than 700000 laparoscopic cholecystectomies are performed annually in the USA, while in the UK more than 70000 are performed. Reported rates vary widely in different European countries, possibly because of differences in medical coding practices.

There are relatively few contraindications to this procedure. They include severe coagulopathy, severe congestive heart failure and chronic obstructive pulmonary disease; patients with either of the last two conditions may not tolerate the pneumoperitoneum needed for a laparoscopic cholecystectomy. Previous upper abdominal surgery may make the procedure difficult. Laparoscopic cholecystectomy can be performed in patients with well-compensated liver cirrhosis, although there is an increased risk of bleeding in some patients. Conversion to an open operation is needed in about 5% of elective laparoscopic cholecystectomies, usually because anatomic landmarks cannot be seen clearly enough.

Most laparoscopic cholecystectomies are completed safely. Overall, the complication rate is 2.5% (comparable to that associated with open cholecystectomy). The main complications include bleeding, wound infection, bile leak and injury to the bile duct. Less common complications include lacerations of the liver and bowel, pneumoperitoneum-related complications, intra-abdominal abscess due to inadvertent spillage of gallstones into the abdominal cavity, and retained CBD stones. The risk of biliary injury during laparoscopic cholecystectomy diminishes as the surgeon acquires experience and expertise.

Medical management. Although laparoscopic cholecystectomy remains the definitive treatment for gallstone disease, selected patients who are unfit for surgery may be candidates for medical therapy.

Bile acid treatment options include ursodeoxycholic acid, which works by forming liquid cholesterol crystals, and chenodeoxycholic acid, which removes cholesterol as micelles. This treatment is most successful for small stones in a normally functioning gallbladder and in the absence of acute cholecystitis. Prolonged treatment (up to 2 years) is usually required. Use of these agents may be limited by cost and side effects, notably diarrhea; the recurrence rate is around 50% after 5 years.

Contact dissolution involves the use of solvents that dissolve gallstones on direct contact, but is now rarely used because of serious complications.

Extracorporeal shock wave lithotripsy may be performed to destroy gallstones. It can be used on multiple stones, but is most effective for a single stone; the selection criteria to improve the results of the treatment are:
• solitary stone
• stone < 2 cm
• normally functioning gallbladder
• non-obstructed cystic duct.

Bile acid treatment is combined with lithotripsy to promote clearance of stone fragments. Common complications of lithotripsy include biliary colic and pain. Less common complications include biliary obstruction, acute pancreatitis and injury to adjacent organs.

Prognosis and follow-up. Asymptomatic gallstones rarely lead to complications and problems. If the gallstones are causing obstruction, they can lead to blockage of the cystic duct with biliary type pain or acute cholecystitis (see below). If the stones are passing in the common bile duct they can further cause obstruction and jaundice, as well as cholangitis (see Chapter 4). Gallbladder cancer is a rare complication of gallbladder stones (see page 32–7).

Acute cholecystitis
Etiology and pathogenesis. Acute cholecystitis caused by gallstones is in most cases due to obstruction of the cystic duct, which results in distension and inflammation of the gallbladder wall, which in turn may result in ischemia and necrosis. Inflammation and stasis may lead to secondary infection of bile. Severe cases may present with sepsis. Acalculous cholecystitis (see below) also occurs, notably as a complication of cardiac surgery or in patients in intensive care units.

Epidemiology and risk factors. Acute cholecystitis is the most frequent complication of gallstones. About 10% of symptomatic gallstone patients will develop acute cholecystitis.

Up to 15% of acute cholecystitis occurs in the absence of gallstones and is called acute acalculous cholecystitis (see page 31). Critically ill patients in intensive care units who are fasting are particularly at risk for developing this variety. The incidence of acute cholecystitis is approximately the same in the USA and Europe. The exact worldwide incidence is not known but will mirror the rates of gallstone disease.

Diagnosis is through laboratory tests and imaging. Figure 3.4 shows a diagnostic algorithm for acute cholecystitis.

Symptoms and signs include pain or tenderness and guarding in the right upper quadrant, nausea and vomiting, fever, fast pulse (tachycardia) and a positive Murphy's sign (transient cessation of breathing due to pain during inspiration while the right upper quadrant is palpated, but not the left upper quadrant). Complications include empyema, perforation of the gallbladder, liver abscess and emphysematous cholecystitis. An inflamed and distended gallbladder may obstruct the main bile duct by pressure from a gallstone causing obstructive jaundice (Mirizzi's syndrome).

Laboratory tests. Leukocytosis and mild elevation in serum bilirubin and transaminases may be present.

Transabdominal ultrasonography is the most useful test for acute cholecystitis as it establishes the presence of gallstones (Figure 3.5). A thickened gallbladder wall (> 4 mm) and pericholecystic fluid are highly suggestive of acute cholecystitis (Figure 3.6). Sonographic Murphy's sign (tenderness over the gallbladder from the ultrasound transducer during imaging) is also diagnostic.

Radionuclide scanning is a useful test if ultrasound is non-diagnostic or inconclusive but there is clinical suspicion of acute cholecystitis. A ^{99}Tc–HIDA (hepatobiliary iminodiacetic acid) scan uses a technetium-labeled analog of iminodiacetic acid. Non-visualization of the gallbladder with visualization of the tracer in the CBD and the small intestine is consistent with cystic duct obstruction. This test is about 95% accurate for the diagnosis of acute cholecystitis.

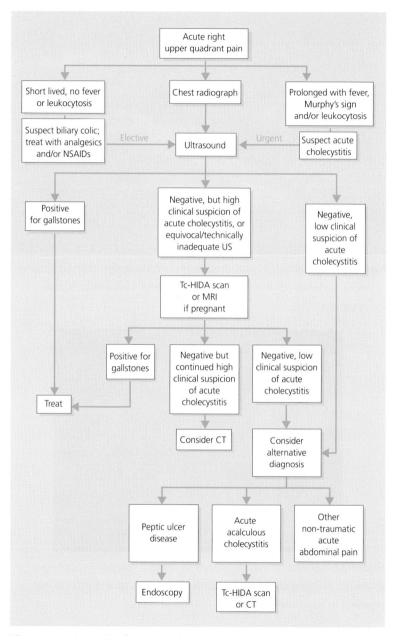

Figure 3.4 Diagnosis of acute cholecystitis. CT, computed tomography, HIDA, hepatobiliary iminodiacetic acid; NSAID, non-steroidal anti-inflammatory drug; US, ultrasonography.

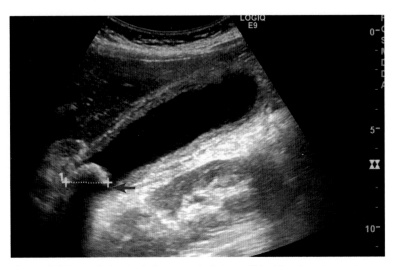

Figure 3.5 Transabdominal ultrasound of the gallbladder showing a stone with characteristic posterior acoustic shadow and surrounding sludge (microlithiasis).

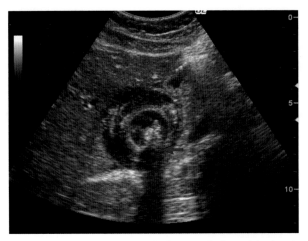

Figure 3.6 Transabdominal ultrasound of acute cholecystitis showing a thickened wall, a small amount of pericholecystic fluid and a stone with posterior acoustic shadowing.

Computed tomography is useful for identifying local complications of acute cholecystitis (Figure 3.7).

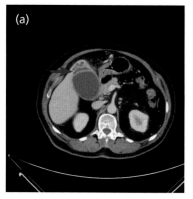 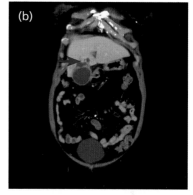

Figure 3.7 CT scan of acute cholecystitis showing an enlarged gallbladder with thickened wall and a liver abscess in the vicinity: (a) axial and (b) coronal sections.

Medical treatment of acute cholecystitis involves:
- nothing by mouth
- intravenous fluids
- intravenous antibiotics
- analgesics.

Surgical treatment. The definitive treatment is cholecystectomy, which is usually performed laparoscopically, although conversion to open cholecystectomy may be needed. Comparative studies of immediate (within 24–48 hours) versus delayed (after 6 weeks) laparoscopic cholecystectomy show similar rates for success, complications and conversion to open procedure. However, early laparoscopic cholecystectomy decreases hospital stay and medical costs. Subtotal cholecystectomy is sometimes needed if there is extensive inflammation and fibrosis around the gallbladder, making dissection more difficult and higher risk.

Prognosis and follow up. Uncomplicated acute cholecystitis has an excellent prognosis, with resolution of symptoms during medical treatment, followed by surgery. Cases complicated by perforation and bile peritonitis have a reserved prognosis, as they require urgent surgery.

Chronic cholecystitis

Etiology and pathogenesis. Gallstones are the causative agent in the majority of patients with chronic cholecystitis. Recurrent or chronic obstruction of the cystic duct results in chronic inflammation of the gallbladder wall, which may lead to a non-functioning gallbladder. There is a small, long-term risk of developing gallbladder cancer.

Epidemiology and risk factors. Chronic cholecystitis is generally caused by repeated milder attacks of acute calculous cholecystitis or by mechanical irritation of the gallbladder wall by gallstones. These cause the wall of the gallbladder to thicken. The gallbladder begins to shrink, and is subsequently less able to concentrate, store and release bile. The disease occurs more often in women than in men and is more common after 40 years of age.

Diagnosis

Symptoms and signs include right upper quadrant and epigastric pain. Pain may be episodic and recurrent without the clinical features of acute cholecystitis, but constant right upper quadrant or epigastric pain is the more usual pattern in patients with chronic cholecystitis. Nausea and vomiting may occur when the pain is severe. Episodic pain may or may not be associated with meals, and right upper quadrant tenderness may or may not be present on physical examination. Common laboratory tests are normal.

Transabdominal ultrasonography is the best test to demonstrate the presence of gallstones. Sludge is often seen in patients who have not eaten for at least a day and may be associated with other intra-abdominal illness; however, it is not itself indicative of gallbladder disease. Thickening of the gallbladder wall may be seen in some patients.

Endoscopic ultrasonography may be used in patients with chronic biliary-type pain who have no gallstones on transabdominal ultrasound. EUS may demonstrate microlithiasis (gallstones ≤ 3 mm and that usually do not cast an acoustic shadow).

Dynamic hepatobiliary iminodiacetic acid scanning may be performed in selected patients with suspected gallbladder dysfunction when no gallstones or microlithiasis can be proven or if the symptoms are unusual. A low gallbladder ejection fraction on gallbladder stimulation (cholecystokinin injection) and scan is consistent with the dysfunctional gallbladder that occurs in chronic cholecystitis. Reproduction of the patient's pain during the test may help establish a biliary cause of pain in atypical cases.

Treatment is by laparoscopic cholecystectomy. Conversion to open cholecystectomy is required in about 5% of patients.

Acalculous cholecystitis

Etiology and pathogenesis. Acalculous cholecystitis is an acute inflammatory condition that occurs in patients without gallstones. Stasis and ischemia are considered to be underlying pathophysiological factors that lead to a local inflammatory response resulting in gallbladder distention. Secondary infection and necrosis of the gallbladder wall can then occur. Acalculous cholecystitis may lead to spontaneous perforation of the gallbladder.

Epidemiology and risk factors. Acalculous cholecystitis is associated with a myriad of clinical conditions and frequently occurs in critically ill patients, with the incidence in this group ranging from 0.5 to 18%. There are many predisposing risk factors (Table 3.2).

TABLE 3.2

Predisposing risk factors for acalculous cholecystitis

• Surgery	• Diabetes mellitus
• Sepsis	• Severe infections
• Shock	• Critical illness managed in the intensive care unit
• Pregnancy	
• Total parenteral nutrition	• AIDS
• Ventilator support	• Bone marrow transplant
• Trauma	• Burns
	• Coronary heart disease

Diagnosis

Symptoms and signs. The usual scenario consists of abdominal pain, fever and leukocytosis in a patient with one of the above predisposing conditions. Diagnosis requires a high index of suspicion. Right upper quadrant tenderness and Murphy's sign may be present, and a palpable mass may be detected in a minority of patients. Jaundice is not uncommon.

Laboratory test results indicative of acalculous cholecystitis include leukocytosis, abnormal transaminases, hyperbilirubinemia and increased alkaline phosphatase levels.

Plain abdominal radiography is useful to identify emphysematous cholecystitis, gas in the gallbladder and free air in the abdomen resulting from a perforated gallbladder.

Transabdominal ultrasonography is the test of choice and can be done at the bedside in critically ill patients. It may reveal thickening of the gallbladder wall with pericholecystic fluid but no gallstones. Perforation of the gallbladder, abscess in the gallbladder fossa or air in the gallbladder wall may also be seen on ultrasound.

Hepatobiliary iminodiacetic acid scanning may be used in selected cases if abdominal ultrasound is inconclusive. Non-visualization of the gallbladder is diagnostic of acute cholecystitis, but false-positive HIDA findings may occur in a variety of conditions.

Computed tomography may show gallbladder inflammation, pericholecystic fluid or empyema of the gallbladder.

Treatment. Patients require intravenous antibiotics. The treatment of choice is cholecystectomy; it may be attempted laparoscopically, but conversion to the open route may be needed. Percutaneous cholecystostomy may be considered as a temporary measure in patients who are too ill to undergo cholecystectomy. The disease has a high mortality, which is influenced significantly by the patient's underlying condition.

Prognosis and follow-up. The prognosis is guarded for patients with acute acalculous cholecystitis. The mortality for critically ill patients reaches up to 50%.

Gallbladder polyps

Etiology and pathogenesis. Gallbladder polyps are seen in about 5% of normal subjects undergoing gallbladder ultrasonography. Differential diagnosis of polypoid lesions of the gallbladder includes cholesterol polyps, adenomyomatosis, inflammatory polyps, adenomas and gallbladder carcinoma.

Cholesterol polyps are the result of abnormal deposition of cholesterol and triglycerides into the gallbladder wall. Adenomyomatosis is characterized by thickening of the muscle in the gallbladder wall with overgrowth of the mucosa. Inflammatory polyps are benign non-neoplastic polyps. Adenomas are epithelial growths that can be precursors to gallbladder cancer.

The major clinical significance relates to the malignant potential of the polyps. Risk factors that increase the chance of malignancy in a gallbladder polyp include:

- size > 1 cm
- presence of gallstones
- age > 60 years
- increase in size on interval imaging.

Epidemiology and risk factors. In a Scandinavian study the prevalence of gallbladder polyps as assessed by ultrasonography in a random population was 4.6% among men and 4.3% among women. The prevalence of polyps was not significantly associated with age, sex, social or weight factors, physical activity, diabetes mellitus, pregnancies, use of exogenous female hormones, alcohol intake or plasma lipids. However, in a Chinese study of more than 60 000 people, the overall prevalence of gallbladder polyps was 6.9%. Male sex, hepatitis B virus infection and cholecystitis were strong risk factors for the formation of gallbladder polyps.

Diagnosis

Symptoms and signs. Most patients with gallbladder polyps are asymptomatic, with discovery usually being incidental on imaging studies, although some patients may present with chronic and recurrent biliary-type pain.

31

Transabdominal ultrasonography. Gallbladder polyps are easily visualized. The size and echo features of the polyp(s) assist in differential diagnosis and determination of malignant potential (> 1 cm in size is significantly associated with presence of malignancy). Cholesterol polyps may be multiple, are usually pedunculated and are hyperechoic, but with no acoustic shadow. Adenomas are usually solitary, sessile and more isoechoic.

Computed tomography is not useful for the detection or differential diagnosis of small gallbladder polyps. It is more useful as a preoperative staging technique if malignancy is suspected in a polypoid lesion of the gallbladder.

Endoscopic ultrasonography is a more precise modality for gallbladder imaging than transabdominal ultrasound, but is more invasive. Data from a few studies show better differentiation of neoplastic and non-neoplastic polyps.

Treatment. Cholecystectomy is indicated for polyps greater than 1 cm, for polyps with associated gallstones and for patients with biliary symptoms.

Solitary sessile polyps that are 5–10 mm in size are more likely to be neoplastic than small, multiple, pedunculated, hyperechoic polyps. Cholecystectomy should be considered if a neoplastic polyp is suspected.

Follow-up. Observation with serial imaging is an option for small polyps that are considered to be at low risk for neoplastic features. Polyps that increase in size on serial imaging are an indication for cholecystectomy.

Gallbladder carcinoma

Etiology and pathogenesis. Chronic gallbladder inflammation is attributed as an etiologic factor in gallbladder cancer along with molecular alterations in *p53* and *K-ras*. Inflammation may occur as a result of gallstones, gallbladder polyps, chronic *Salmonella* infection, congenital biliary cysts, abnormal pancreaticobiliary duct junction, carcinogen exposure and certain drugs. There are molecular differences between gallbladder cancers associated with gallstones and those with an abnormal pancreaticobiliary junction.

Epidemiology and risk factors. Gallbladder carcinoma is the fifth most common gastrointestinal (GI) cancer in the USA and is the most common GI cancer in Native Americans. Incidence and mortality are very high in certain Latin American countries, especially Chile.

Risk factors for gallbladder cancer are outlined in Table 3.3. The majority of gallbladder cancers are adenocarcinomas.

Diagnosis

Symptoms and signs include abdominal pain (usually in the right upper quadrant), weight loss, anorexia, nausea and vomiting, fever, obstructive jaundice (from invasion of the bile duct) and duodenal obstruction.

The clinical presentation may mimic acute cholecystitis, chronic cholecystitis or biliary obstruction due to other benign or malignant causes.

Physical examination. Patients may have right upper quadrant tenderness and a palpable mass in the right upper quadrant.

Laboratory tests. Laboratory abnormalities will depend on the clinical presentation of, for example, acute or chronic cholecystitis, biliary obstruction, anorexia, weight loss or malaise without clinical evidence of cholecystitis or biliary obstruction.

TABLE 3.3

Risk factors for gallbladder cancer

- Gallstones
- Choledochal cysts
- Porcelain gallbladder
- Gallbladder polyps
- Anomalous pancreatic biliary junction
- Chronic *Salmonella*-type gallbladder infection

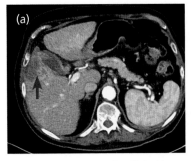 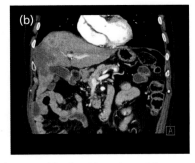

Figure 3.8 CT scan of gallbladder carcinoma with direct invasion of the liver parenchyma and liver metastases: (a) axial and (b) coronal sections.

Transabdominal ultrasonography is the usual initial method for imaging the gallbladder. Ultrasonographic findings of gallbladder cancer include a mass in the gallbladder, significant thickening or irregularity of the gallbladder wall and evidence of loss of interface with the liver or invasion of the liver.

The sensitivity of transabdominal ultrasound for detecting or suggesting the diagnosis of gallbladder cancer may be more than 70%, but its accuracy for regional and distant staging is limited – 50% or less.

Computed tomography is useful for staging to detect liver invasion, lymphadenopathy and distant metastases (Figure 3.8).

MRI with MR cholangiopancreatography may be useful in mapping the extent of a tumor. Vascular encasement, particularly of the portal vein, lymphadenopathy and the complete biliary tree can be visualized.

Endoscopic retrograde cholangiopancreatography or percutaneous transhepatic cholangiography are not needed routinely unless the patient presents with obstructive jaundice requiring biliary decompression, without an obvious diagnosis of gallbladder cancer.

Endoscopic ultrasonography is useful in regional staging of gallbladder cancer associated with lymph-node metastases and vascular invasion. It may also be helpful in differentiating between benign and malignant gallbladder polyps.

Treatment. Staging of gallbladder cancer is shown in Table 3.4. Some surgeons recommend a staging laparoscopy before attempting surgical resection of known or suspected gallbladder cancer.

TABLE 3.4

TNM staging of gallbladder cancer

TX:	Primary tumor cannot be assessed
T0:	No evidence of primary tumor
Tis:	Carcinoma in situ
T1	Tumor invades lamina propria (T1a) or muscle layer (T1b)
T2	Tumor invades perimuscular connective tissue
T3	Tumor perforates the serosa and/or directly invades the liver and/or one other adjacent organ or structure, such as stomach, duodenum, colon, pancreas, omentum or extrahepatic bile ducts
T4	Tumor invades main portal vein or hepatic artery, or invades multiple extrahepatic organs or structures
Nx	Regional lymph nodes cannot be assessed
N0	No regional lymph-node metastases
N1	Regional lymph-node metastases to nodes along the cystic duct, common bile duct, hepatic artery and/or portal vein
N2	Metastases to periaortic, pericaval, superior mesenteric artery, and/or celiac artery lymph nodes
Mx	Distant metastases cannot be assessed
M0	No distant metastases
M1	Distant metastases

Stage grouping

I	T1, N0, M0
II	T2, N0, M0
IIIA	T3, N0, M0
IIIB	T1-T3, N1, M0
IVA	T4, N0-1, M0
IVB	any T, N2, M0 or any T, any N, M1

TNM, primary tumor, regional nodes, metastasis.

T1 lesions are usually found incidentally during cholecystectomy and are associated with a 5-year survival rate in 85% of patients. T1b patients have increased risk of lymph-node metastases. Many surgeons prefer reoperation with radical resection to maximize survival. T2 lesions should also be considered for radical resection. Radical resection with an extended cholecystectomy should be performed for stages II and III. Radical surgery for T3 or T4 disease has become more popular and may involve hepatic, pancreatic, duodenal and colonic resection. A hepatic lobectomy may be needed for anatomic reasons in some patients.

Treatment of unresectable disease with palliative chemotherapy and radiation therapy should be considered. Gemcitabine, cisplatin and 5-fluorouracil may be used for palliation, but only limited success has been achieved, and there are no firm recommendations. Radiation therapy using external-beam radiation has had limited effect in patients with unresectable tumors. Palliation for jaundice and bowel obstruction may involve surgical or endoscopic methods.

Key points – diseases of the gallbladder

- The prevalence of gallstones is greater in people over 40 years of age, and women are at higher risk than men.
- Transabdominal ultrasound is the imaging test of choice, with an accuracy of over 95%, for the diagnosis of gallstones in either acute or chronic cholecystitis. A ^{99}Tc–HIDA (hepatobiliary iminodiacetic acid) scan is 95% accurate for the diagnosis of acute cholecystitis.
- Acalculous cholecystitis may occur in critically ill patients; the diagnosis requires a high index of suspicion.
- Patients with gallbladder polyps more than 1 cm in size should be considered for cholecystectomy owing to the increased risk of malignancy.
- Gallbladder cancer is the most common gastrointestinal cancer in Native Americans in the USA and also has a very high incidence in certain Latin American countries, particularly Chile.

Prognosis and follow-up. Prognosis and survival depend on the stage of the disease: nearly 100% for T1a, 75% for T1b, 50–60% for T2 and 25–63% for stages IIA and IIB. Most patients who have unresectable tumors at the time of diagnosis have a 5-year survival of less than 15–20%.

Future trends

- Improved understanding of the carcinogenesis pathways of gallbladder cancer and its precursor lesions.
- Improved non-invasive and minimally invasive imaging techniques.
- Multimodal treatment approaches for gallbladder cancer.
- Novel biological therapies.
- Cancer vaccines and gene therapy.

Key references

Caddy GR, Tham TC. Gallstone disease: Symptoms, diagnosis and endoscopic management of common bile duct stones. *Best Pract Res Clin Gastroenterol* 2006;20:1085–101.

Carroll PJ, Gibson D, El-Faedy O et al. Surgeon-performed ultrasound at the bedside for the detection of appendicitis and gallstones: systematic review and meta-analysis. *Am J Surg* 2013;205:102–8.

Catalano OA, Sahani DV, Kalva SP et al. MR imaging of the gallbladder: a pictorial essay. *Radiographics* 2008;28:135–55;quiz 324.

Chijiiwa K, Nakano K, Ueda J et al. Surgical treatment of patients with T2 gallbladder carcinoma invading the subserosal layer. *J Am Coll Surg* 2001;192:600–7.

Everhart JE, Yeh F, Lee ET et al. Prevalence of gallbladder disease in American Indian populations: Findings from the Strong Heart Study. *Hepatology* 2002;35: 1507–12.

Fuks D, Cossé C, Régimbeau JM. Antibiotic therapy in acute calculous cholecystitis. *J Visc Surg* 2013;150:3–8.

Gore RM, Yaghmai V, Newmark GM et al. Imaging benign and malignant disease of the gallbladder. *Radiol Clin North Am* 2002;40:1307–23.

Gurusamy KS, Davidson BR. Gallstones. *BMJ* 2014;348:g2669.

Habib FA, Kolachalam RB, Khilnani R et al. Role of laparoscopic cholecystectomy in the management of gangrenous cholecystitis. *Am J Surg* 2001;181:71–5.

Kaura SH, Haghighi M, Matza BW et al. Comparison of CT and MRI findings in the differentiation of acute from chronic cholecystitis. *Clin Imaging* 2013;37:687–91.

Misra S, Chaturvedi A, Misra NC, Sharma ID. Carcinoma of the gallbladder. *Lancet Oncol* 2003;4:167–76.

Pandey M, Sood BP, Shukla RC, Aryya NC. Carcinoma of the gallbladder: role of sonography in diagnosis and staging. *J Clin Ultrasound* 2000;28:227–32.

Rubin RA, Kowalski TE, Khandelwal M, Malet PF. Ursodiol for hepatobiliary disorders. *Ann Intern Med* 1994;121:207–18.

Schmidt M, Dumot JA, Søreide O, Søndenaa K. *Scand J Gastroenterol* 2012;47:1257–65.

Sugiyama M, Atomi Y, Yamato T. Endoscopic ultrasonography for differential diagnosis of polypoid gall bladder lesions: Analysis in surgical and follow up series. *Gut* 2000;46:250–4.

Terzi C, Sokmen S, Seckin S et al. Polypoid lesions of the gallbladder: Report of 100 cases with special reference to operative indications. *Surgery* 2000;127:622–7.

4　Bile duct stone disease (choledocholithiasis)

Etiology and pathogenesis

Stones within the common bile duct (CBD) are usually formed in the gallbladder and pass on to the CBD. They may be of the cholesterol or hard black-pigmented type (see Chapter 3). However, primary stones formed within the bile duct are commonly of the soft brown-pigmented type; they are promoted by stasis. Older adults with larger CBDs or with periampullary diverticula, as well as patients with recurrent or chronic biliary tract infections, may be at greater risk for developing primary stones in the bile duct.

CBD stones are the most frequent cause of extrahepatic obstructive jaundice, generating an increased risk of severe complications, including acute cholangitis or pancreatitis. Cholangitis can occur concurrently with choledocholithiasis; it may be acute or chronic and is caused by at least partial obstruction to bile flow.

Epidemiology and risk factors

Around 10% of younger patients with stones in the gallbladder have CBD stones at the time of cholecystectomy, rising with age to around 20%. The exact prevalence and incidence of bile duct stones is not known.

Diagnosis

Symptoms and signs include right upper quadrant pain/tenderness, jaundice, fever, clay-colored stools and dark urine. Symptoms and signs of concomitant acute cholangitis include pain and tenderness in the right upper quadrant, jaundice and fever spikes (> 38°C) with chills (Charcot's triad). Patients with severe or suppurative cholangitis are severely ill, with septicemia, shock and mental confusion.

Laboratory tests may reveal elevated serum levels of bilirubin, alkaline phosphatase, γ-glutamyltransferase, aspartate aminotransferase and alanine aminotransferase, although these tests may occasionally be normal in patients with CBD stones. Leukocytosis is seen in patients with cholangitis. Increased amylase or lipase are present in patients with acute biliary pancreatitis.

Transabdominal ultrasound is non-invasive and is generally the first imaging modality used when a stone in the CBD is suspected. Its sensitivity for detection of a dilated bile duct is up to 90%, and even higher in jaundiced patients. However, its sensitivity for detection of stones in the CBD is lower, about 25–80%, depending on the examiner's experience and the size of the bile duct (Figure 4.1).

Endoscopic ultrasonography (EUS) is a minimally invasive endoscopic imaging modality for CBD stones with an accuracy of around 98% (Figure 4.2). It can be performed in a combined session with therapeutic endoscopic retrograde cholangiopancreatography (ERCP) to achieve diagnosis and stone removal.

Magnetic resonance cholangiopancreatography (MRCP) is a non-invasive technique for imaging the extra- and intrahepatic biliary system with a sensitivity of 93% and specificity of 94% (Figure 4.3). Contraindications include claustrophobia and implanted metal devices and fragments. MRCP is a useful, non-invasive and reliable test for CBD stones. MRCP and EUS generally have comparable high accuracy; however, for small stones less than 6 mm in diameter, EUS may be more accurate.

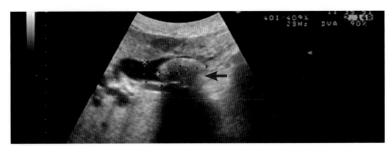

Figure 4.1 Transabdominal ultrasonogram showing a dilated common bile duct (CBD) with a large stone of 3.6 cm in the terminal part of the CBD.

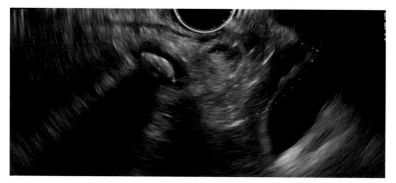

Figure 4.2 Endoscopic ultrasonogram showing a non-dilated common bile duct with a small stone of 4 mm, with characteristic posterior acoustic shadow.

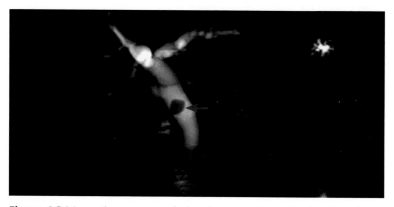

Figure 4.3 Magnetic resonance cholangiopancreatography showing a large stone in a dilated common bile duct.

Computed tomography cholangiography involves imaging the biliary ductal system after injection of contrast medium. The accuracy for CBD stones is around 85%, less than for EUS and MRCP.

Endoscopic retrograde cholangiopancreatography is accurate in more than 90% of patients but should be performed only with the intent for therapeutic intervention (Figure 4.4). ERCP is more invasive than other imaging modalities, with risks that include acute pancreatitis (about 5%), bleeding and perforation. Intraductal ultrasound during ERCP has a similar accuracy and is marginally superior to ERCP alone.

41

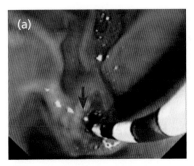 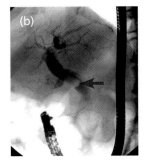

Figure 4.4 Endoscopic retrograde cholangiopancreatography in a Billroth II patient (see Figure 5.4; Table 5.2), showing a 10 mm common bile duct (CBD) stone after retrograde cannulation of the CBD. (a) Endoscopic image of the catheter cannulating the ampulla and (b) radiological image of the bile duct with the stone after retrograde contrast injection.

These diagnostic ERCP techniques are invasive and should generally not be used in preference to conventional EUS or MRCP.

Intraoperative cholangiography is performed at the time of cholecystectomy to detect the presence of CBD stones. It is performed routinely at some institutions, whereas others perform it when there is suspicion of retained CBD stones. In an analysis of more than 4000 patients undergoing laparoscopic cholecystectomy, 4% of patients were found to have stones in the CBD, but small stones do sometimes pass spontaneously from the CBD into the duodenum.

Choosing the right diagnostic test

Suspected choledocholithiasis and intact gallbladder. When there is high suspicion for the presence of a CBD stone on the basis of symptoms, signs, laboratory tests and abdominal ultrasound, one may proceed directly to ERCP, but in general EUS or MRCP should be performed as a prelude. If the preliminary examination proves negative then a cholecystectomy may be undertaken with the option of performing an intraoperative cholangiogram.

Suspected choledocholithiasis after cholecystectomy. If there is high suspicion for CBD stones, one may proceed directly to ERCP, but again, in general, the diagnosis should first be confirmed by EUS or

MRCP. Patients for whom the suspicion of CBD stones is low may be observed clinically for a while before initiating any investigation involving EUS or MRCP.

Medical treatment

Any patient with obstructive jaundice, irrespective of the cause, is at risk of increased bleeding owing to malabsorption of vitamin K (bile-acid-dependent), which is required by the liver to synthesize clotting factors II, VII, IX and X. Thus, the prothrombin time, partial thromboplastin time and international normalized ratio need to be checked in all patients. Fresh frozen plasma may be required to correct clotting immediately. All patients with abnormal clotting parameters will need vitamin supplementation by parenteral injection and/or absorbable modified vitamin K by mouth.

Patients with acute cholangitis exhibiting signs of Charcot's triad usually respond to intravenous fluids and antibiotics, but need subsequent clearance of CBD obstruction. Treatment with intravenous fluids and antibiotics may have to be supplemented by intensive care and vasopressors in severe or suppurative cholangitis.

Endoscopic treatment

Endoscopic biliary decompression by ERCP with sphincterotomy allows endoscopic extraction of stones from the CBD. If ERCP clears all stones from the CBD, the patient can then undergo laparoscopic cholecystectomy. Some patients may require more than one attempt by ERCP to clear all stones from the CBD. A plastic stent is sometimes placed in the bile duct during ERCP to achieve biliary drainage if it is not possible to remove all the stones and further attempts should be planned. Large stones may require endoscopic lithotripsy during

In acute cholangitis patients, ERCP must be performed as an emergency and, if it is unsuccessful, radiological biliary intervention is required. Surgical intervention is associated with a high mortality and should be undertaken only when other methods have failed.

ERCP with or without cholangioscopy or extracorporeal shock wave lithotripsy in combination with ERCP.

Clearance of all stones from the CBD through ERCP is possible in more than 95% of patients. ERCP with sphincterotomy is also useful for patients who have recently undergone a cholecystectomy and present with retained CBD stones.

Complications of ERCP include pancreatitis, perforation, bleeding and cholangitis in about 5% of patients. The risk of cholangitis after ERCP is increased if ERCP is attempted but biliary drainage is not achieved. Alternative radiological and surgical methods for biliary decompression in acutely ill patients with biliary obstruction should be readily available.

Surgical treatment

Cholecystectomy is recommended after ERCP with sphincterotomy and bile duct stone clearance, in order to prevent recurrence of biliary symptoms and biliary colic.

Surgical exploration of the CBD may be needed for patients with stones that could not be cleared by ERCP. This is, however, a rare event in high volume ERCP centers. Another indication for surgical CBD exploration includes stones discovered during intraoperative cholangiography. Laparoscopic CBD exploration is performed through either the cystic duct or a choledochotomy (requiring postoperative T-tube drainage). This approach is successful in clearing CBD stones in more then 90% of cases.

Open CBD procedures are rarely performed any more but may occasionally be required when other non-surgical or laparoscopic methods are unsuccessful or impossible.

Future trends

Future developments are likely to include:
• more widespread application of non-invasive and minimally invasive imaging with MRCP and EUS
• more clear-cut guidelines on use of various imaging modalities for detection of bile duct stones
• development of video cholangioscopy leading to direct and easy visualization of the bile duct for diagnosis and therapy.

Key points – bile duct stone disease (choledocholithiasis)

- Around 10–20% of patients with stones in the gallbladder have common bile duct (CBD) stones at the time of cholecystectomy (the prevalence rises with age).
- Transabdominal ultrasound is 25–80% accurate for detection of CBD stones, depending on the experience of the examiner.
- Endoscopic ultrasonography and magnetic resonance cholangiopancreatography are accurate tests for detection of CBD stones and should generally precede endoscopic retrograde cholangiopancreatography (ERCP), unless the clinical signs and symptoms and transabdominal ultrasound findings make therapeutic ERCP inevitable.
- Clearance of all stones from the CBD via ERCP is possible in more than 95% of patients.
- Biliary decompression, preferably by endoscopic or radiologic means, is critical in severe suppurative cholangitis with choledocholithiasis.

Key references

Eisen GM, Dominitz JA, Faigel DO et al. An annotated algorithm for the evaluation of choledocholithiasis. *Gastrointest Endosc* 2001;53:864–6.

Ko CW, Lee SP. Epidemiology and natural history of common bile duct stones and prediction of disease. *Gastrointest Endosc* 2002;56(suppl 6):S165–9.

Napoléon B, Dumortier J, Keriven-Souquet O et al. Do normal findings at biliary endoscopic ultrasonography obviate the need for endoscopic retrograde cholangiography in patients with suspicion of common bile duct stone? A prospective follow-up study of 238 patients. *Endoscopy* 2003;35:411–15.

NIH state-of-the-science statement on endoscopic retrograde cholangiopancreatography (ERCP) for diagnosis and therapy. NIH *Consens State Sci Statements* 2002;19:1–26.

Rickes S, Treiber G, Mönkemüller K et al. Impact of the operator's experience on value of high-resolution transabdominal ultrasound in the diagnosis of choledocholithiasis: a prospective comparison using endoscopic retrograde cholangiography as the gold standard. *Scand J Gastroenterol* 2006;41:838–43.

Scheiman JM, Carlos RC, Barnett JL et al. Can endoscopic ultrasound or magnetic resonance cholangiopancreatography replace ERCP in patients with suspected biliary disease? A prospective trial and cost analysis. *Am J Gastroenterol* 2001;96:2900–4.

Tse F, Yuan Y. Early routine endoscopic retrograde cholangiopancreatography strategy versus early conservative management strategy in acute gallstone pancreatitis. *Cochrane Database Syst Rev* 2012;5:CD009779.

van Erpecum KJ. Gallstone disease. Complications of bile-duct stones: Acute cholangitis and pancreatitis. *Best Pract Res Clin Gastroenterol* 2006;20:1139–52.

Yusuf TE, Bhutani MS. Role of endoscopic ultrasonography in diseases of the extrahepatic biliary system. *J Gastroenterol Hepatol* 2004;19:243–50.

Cholangiocarcinoma

Etiology and pathogenesis. Bile duct cancer or cholangiocarcinoma may arise in the intra- or extrahepatic biliary system. The bifurcation of the hepatic duct (hilum) is the most common site for cholangiocarcinomas (Klatskin tumor). Adenocarcinoma is the most common histological type; molecular changes include the expression of mutant *p53* and *K-ras*.

The overall pathophysiology of cholangiocarcinoma is poorly understood. Mutations leading to cholangiocarcinoma occur in a background of chronic inflammation, leading to proliferation of mutated cells and angiogenesis.

Epidemiology and risk factors. Cholangiocarcinoma occurs predominantly in patients aged 50–70 years and is more common in men than women. Risk factors for cholangiocarcinoma are shown in Table 5.1.

TABLE 5.1

Risk factors for cholangiocarcinoma in order of prevalence

- Primary sclerosing cholangitis
- Choledochal cysts
- Hepatolithiasis
- Liver flukes
- Oriental cholangiohepatitis
- Toxins (thorium dioxide contrast medium, rubber and other chemicals)
- Biliary papillomatosis
- Bile duct adenoma

Diagnosis

Symptoms and signs include obstructive jaundice, pruritus, right upper quadrant pain, weight loss, fever, acholic (pale) stools, dark urine and hepatomegaly. A right upper quadrant mass may be present.

Laboratory tests may show increased levels of bilirubin, aspartate aminotransferase, alanine aminotransferase, alkaline phosphatase and γ-glutamyltransferase. The serum tumor markers carcinoembryonic antigen and cancer antigen 19.9 are usually elevated; however, they may also indicate other types of tumor, and can be mildly or moderately elevated in benign biliary obstruction.

Transabdominal ultrasonography or CT should be undertaken as the initial diagnostic step in patients with suspected pancreaticobiliary cancer (Figure 5.1). Transabdominal ultrasound indicates the level of biliary obstruction and sometimes the tumor mass itself (Figure 5.2).

Computed tomography will usually show the position and extent of a hilar cholangiocarcinoma along with a dilated intrahepatic biliary system, with a non-dilated extrahepatic biliary tree and a non-dilated gallbladder. A CT scan of a distal bile duct cancer will show dilation of the intra- and extrahepatic biliary systems and the gallbladder.

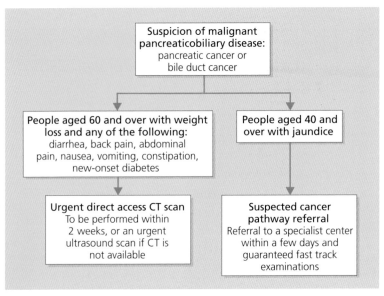

Figure 5.1 Diagnosis of pancreaticobiliary cancer.

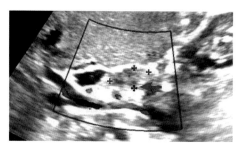

Figure 5.2 Transabdominal ultrasound showing a dilated common bile duct (CBD) with a hypoechoic mass in the terminal part of the CBD, confirmed as a distal cholangiocarcinoma.

CT scans have limited ability to determine the resectability and extent of a tumor and often need to be supplemented by additional techniques, such as positron-emission tomography (PET), to enhance their accuracy. PET scans have a pooled sensitivity and specificity of over 80%, especially for intrahepatic or hilar cholangiocarcinoma. The radiation exposure associated with a PET–CT scan should always be considered.

Magnetic resonance cholangiopancreatography may provide supplementary definition of both the tumor and extent of biliary obstruction (Figure 5.3).

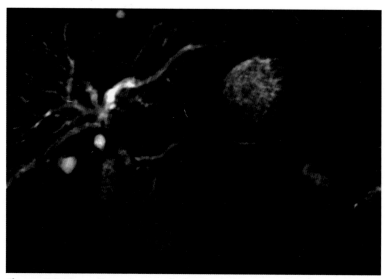

Figure 5.3 Magnetic resonance cholangiopancreatography, showing hilar obstruction and marked dilation of the intrahepatic bile ducts in a proximal cholangiocarcinoma (Klatskin tumor).

Endoscopic retrograde cholangiopancreatography or percutaneous transhepatic cholangiography is performed to obtain a diagnosis by brush cytology and permit temporary or permanent biliary decompression by means of a plastic or metal mesh stent, respectively.

Other imaging modalities include endoscopic ultrasonography (EUS) and laparoscopic ultrasound, which may be useful adjuncts for establishing and defining the location and extent of a tumor. EUS fine needle aspiration (EUS-FNA) is another option; it may be useful preoperatively to establish a definitive diagnosis, and recent data suggest that it may not adversely affect overall survival.

Staging and classification. Hilar cholangiocarcinoma is classified according to the Bismuth classification (Figure 5.4; Table 5.2).

Treatment. A surgical cure is possible in only a small proportion of patients. The type of operation depends on the location of the tumor.
- A distal cholangiocarcinoma is treated with a partial duodenopancreatectomy (Whipple's procedure).

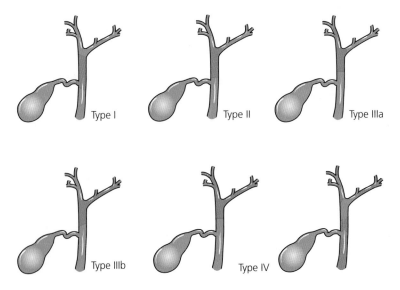

Figure 5.4 Bismuth classification of perihilar cholangiocarcinoma (see also Table 5.2). (See De Groen et al. *N Engl J Med* 1999;341:1368–78.)

TABLE 5.2

The Bismuth classification and staging of perihilar cholangiocarcinoma

Type	Description of tumor (Figure 5.4)
I	Confined to the common hepatic duct
II	Involves the hepatic bifurcation but not the secondary intrahepatic ducts
IIIa	Involves the hepatic bifurcation and the right secondary intrahepatic ducts
IIIb	Involves the hepatic bifurcation and the left secondary intrahepatic ducts
IV	Involves the hepatic bifurcation and extends to both left and right secondary intrahepatic ducts

Stage	
IA	Tumor involves only the bile duct
IB	Tumor involves periductal tissues
IIA	Locally advanced tumor that is devoid of lymph-node metastases
IIB	Locally advanced tumor with adjacent lymph-node metastases
III	Unresectable, locally advanced tumor
IV	Tumor with distant metastases

- A hilar lesion may be treated by local resection but usually requires a partial hepatic resection; in either case a hepaticojejunostomy is required to restore continuity of the biliary-enteric tract.
- Intrahepatic lesions are treated with hepatic resection.
  Preoperative stenting for alleviation of biliary obstruction may avoid deterioration of liver function, but increases the risk of cholangitis and other complications following resection, especially in hilar lesions.

The 5-year survival after surgical resection varies from 10% to 40%.

51

Palliation of unresectable tumors. Biliary drainage may be achieved in unresectable disease with stents placed endoscopically or radiologically. Stents may be plastic (removable) or expandable metallic stents (non-removable). The method and choice of stent insertion depends on the location of the tumor, local expertise and whether unresectability has been clearly determined at the time of stent insertion.

The value of chemotherapy or radiation therapy in prolonging survival has not been adequately established. Randomized studies using local photodynamic or radiofrequency ablation therapy have demonstrated prolonged biliary patency and survival.

Other bile duct tumors

Table 5.3 lists the various bile duct tumors.

Biliary papillomatosis presents as tumorous papillary growths of the bile duct epithelium, which are usually diffuse and multiple. A large amount of mucus is produced by the abnormal biliary epithelium,

TABLE 5.3

Tumors of the bile duct

- Cholangiocarcinoma
- Biliary papilloma
- Biliary cystadenoma
- Non-Hodgkin's lymphoma
- MALT lymphoma
- Carcinoid tumor
- Granular cell tumor
- Teratoma
- Adenoma
- Adenomyoma
- Metastases

MALT, mucosa-associated lymphoid tissue.

causing biliary obstruction with resultant cholestatic jaundice and cholangitis. A possible association between Caroli's disease and biliary papillomatosis has been reported.

Biliary cystadenoma is a rare tumor. Malignant degeneration does occur, but very little is known of the risk for this. Because of the risk for malignancy and recurrence, surgical treatment encompassing resection or complete enucleation is recommended.

Lymphoma of the bile duct. Primary non-Hodgkin's lymphoma may arise from the bile duct. Jaundice may occur due to a variety of causes, including direct hepatic involvement or compression of the bile ducts by lymph nodes, as well as tumor-related hemolysis. This tumor can occur between the first and seventh decades of life. The most common lymphoma subtype pattern is large-cell lymphoma. Treatment is variable and includes a combination of chemotherapy, radiation and surgery.

Future trends

Future developments are likely to include:

- improved understanding of risk factors and etiopathogenesis, especially for cholangiocarcinoma, which might be induced by chronic biliary inflammation, changing growth factor and proinflammatory cytokine expression patterns
- improved imaging for preoperative diagnosis (e.g. PET and EUS-FNA)
- better selection of patients with hilar cholangiocarcinoma for liver transplantation
- molecular markers for improved preoperative diagnosis, prognostication and treatment selection
- novel biological therapies, cancer vaccines and gene therapy
- bioabsorbable stents for palliation, in addition to other new and improved local treatments, such as photodynamic therapy, high-intensity focused ultrasonography, etc.
- improved methods for minimally invasive pain control and palliation.

Key points – bile duct tumors

- Bifurcation of the hepatic duct is the most common site for cholangiocarcinoma.
- Primary sclerosing cholangitis is the major risk factor for the development of cholangiocarcinoma.
- Benign biliary obstruction may increase cancer antigen 19.9 levels.
- Biliary papillomatosis lesions are diffuse and multiple, with the abnormal biliary epithelium producing a large amount of mucus.
- Rare tumors include biliary cystadenoma and primary non-Hodgkin's lymphoma.

Key references

American Society for Gastrointestinal Endoscopy Standards of Practice Committee, Anderson MA, Appalaneni V et al. The role of endoscopy in the evaluation and treatment of patients with biliary neoplasia. *Gastrointest Endosc* 2013;77:167–74.

Annunziata S, Caldarella C, Pizzuto DA et al. Diagnostic accuracy of fluorine-18-fluorodeoxyglucose positron emission tomography in the evaluation of the primary tumor in patients with cholangiocarcinoma: a meta-analysis. *Biomed Res Int* 2014;2014:247693.

Burke EC, Jarnagin WR, Hochwald SN et al. Hilar cholangiocarcinoma: patterns of spread, the importance of hepatic resection for curative operation, and a presurgical clinical staging system. *Ann Surg* 1998;228:385–94.

Cameron JL, Pitt HA, Zinner MJ et al. Management of proximal cholangiocarcinoma by surgical resection and radiotherapy. *Am J Surg* 1990;159:91–7(discussion 97–8).

El Chafic AH, Dewitt J, Leblanc JK et al. Impact of preoperative endoscopic ultrasound-guided fine needle aspiration on postoperative recurrence and survival in cholangiocarcinoma patients. *Endoscopy* 2013;45:883–9.

Joo YE, Park CH, Lee WS et al. Primary non-Hodgkin's lymphoma of the common bile duct presenting as obstructive jaundice. *J Gastroenterol* 2004;39:692–6.

Klempnauer J, Ridder GJ, von Wasielewski R et al. Resectional surgery of hilar cholangiocarcinoma: a multivariate analysis of prognostic factors. *J Clin Oncol* 1997;15: 947–54.

Koffron A, Rao S, Ferrario M, Abecassis M. Intrahepatic biliary cystadenoma: role of cyst fluid analysis and surgical management in the laparascopic era. *Surgery* 2004;136:926–36.

Levy MJ, Heimbach JK, Gores GJ. Endoscopic ultrasound staging of cholangiocarcinoma. *Curr Opin Gastroenterol* 2012;28:244–52.

Lillemoe KD, Cameron JL. Surgery for hilar cholangiocarcinoma: the Johns Hopkins approach. *J Hepatobiliary Pancreat Surg* 2000;7:115–21.

Nagino M, Nimura Y, Kamiya J et al. Segmental liver resections for hilar cholangiocarcinoma. *Hepatogastroenterology* 1998; 45:7–13.

Ruys AT, van Beem BE, Engelbrecht MR. Radiological staging in patients with hilar cholangiocarcinoma: a systematic review and meta-analysis. *Br J Radiol* 2012;85:1255–62.

Todoroki T, Kawamoto T, Koike N et al. Radical resection of hilar bile duct carcinoma and predictors of survival. *Br J Surg* 2000;87:306–13.

Tsao JI, Nimura Y, Kamiya J et al. Management of hilar cholangiocarcinoma: comparison of an American and a Japanese experience. *Ann Surg* 2000;232: 166–74.

Ustundag Y, Bayraktar Y. Cholangiocarcinoma: a compact review of the literature. *World J Gastroenterol* 2008;14:6458–66.

Zabron A, Edwards RJ, Khan SA. The challenge of cholangiocarcinoma: dissecting the molecular mechanisms of an insidious cancer. *Dis Model Mech* 2013;6:281–92.

Cysts

Etiology and pathogenesis. There is limited information regarding the etiology and pathogenesis of biliary cysts, and it is likely that the pathogenesis differs between various cysts. Abnormal pancreaticobiliary junctions may play a role in some, while in others a genetic or environmental predisposition may be important.

Cysts of the biliary tree can be congenital or acquired. Congenital cysts may be diagnosed in the prenatal period and there may be a familial occurrence. Cysts involving the biliary tree may be isolated or multiple, and dilation of the biliary tree can be intrahepatic or extrahepatic. More than 70% of patients with choledochal cysts have an abnormal pancreaticobiliary junction, with a long common channel.

Epidemiology and risk factors. The incidence in Western countries varies from 1 in 100 000 to 1 in 150 000. Biliary cysts are more common in East Asian countries. The prevalence is at least threefold higher in women than in men. Biliary cysts are associated with an increased risk for cholangiocarcinoma.

Diagnosis

Symptoms and signs. The classic triad of pain, jaundice and an abdominal mass is seen in only 10% of patients and is most common in infants, who may also present with raised bilirubin or failure to thrive. Common symptoms in adults include chronic intermittent abdominal pain, intermittent jaundice and acute cholangitis. Less common manifestations include pancreatitis, biliary lithiasis and intraperitoneal rupture.

Transabdominal ultrasonography, MRI or CT may suggest the diagnosis.

Magnetic resonance cholangiopancreatography (MRCP) allows non-invasive preoperative evaluation of the biliary tree.

Endoscopic ultrasonography (EUS) is useful for extrahepatic biliary cysts, to delineate the anatomy and to rule out stones or a mass within the dilated duct.

Cholangiography is generally considered the best method for the evaluation and definition of cysts, and for identifying associated stones or malignancy. The cholangiogram may be performed endoscopically, percutaneously or intraoperatively.

Classification of biliary cysts is shown in Table 6.1.

TABLE 6.1 **Classification of biliary cysts**		
Type I	Cystic or fusiform dilation of the extrahepatic biliary tree (most common)	
Type II	Supraduodenal diverticulum of the extrahepatic biliary duct	
Type III	Intraduodenal diverticulum or cystic dilation of the intraduodenal portion (choledochocele)	
Type IVA	Multiple cysts in the extrahepatic and intrahepatic ducts	
Type IVB	Multiple extrahepatic cysts without intrahepatic involvement	
Type V	Isolated or multiple cystic dilations of the intrahepatic biliary tree without extrahepatic involvement	

CBD, common bile duct; CD, cystic duct; CHD, common hepatic duct; D, duodenum; GB, gallbladder; LHD, left hepatic duct; PD, pancreatic duct; RHD, right hepatic duct; SoO, sphincter of Oddi.

Treatment. Type I/II choledochal cysts are treated with cholecystectomy, resection of the extrahepatic biliary duct and hepaticojejunostomy. Type III cysts may be treated endoscopically. Type IV cysts should be resected. Hepatic lobectomy may be considered for intrahepatic cysts limited to one lobe (type V). Stenosis of the hepaticojejunostomy with its sequelae is the most common long-term complication of surgery. Surgery decreases but does not eliminate the risk of cancer.

Caroli's disease

Etiology and pathogenesis. Caroli's disease is a congenital condition characterized by multiple segmental dilations of the intrahepatic bile duct. Stagnation of bile leads to cholelithiasis, and patients have an increased risk for cholangiocarcinoma.

Familial cases have been described, and the gene responsible has been mapped to chromosome 6. It is commonly associated with congenital hepatic fibrosis and may also be associated with renal cysts.

The pathogenesis of Caroli's disease is poorly understood and may be related to ductal plate malformation in the biliary tree. This disease belongs to a group of hepatic fibropolycystic diseases and is a hepatic manifestation of autosomal recessive polycystic kidney disease.

Epidemiology and risk factors. This is a rare disease that is generally transmitted in an autosomal recessive manner. It is more commonly diagnosed in Asia, particularly in young people (younger than 22 years). The disease affects about 1 in 1 million people.

Diagnosis

Symptoms and signs include bacterial cholangitis, hepatic abscess and portal hypertension, leading to varices and ascites. Pruritus may be present and there may be intermittent abdominal pain.

Laboratory tests reveal elevated serum levels of alkaline phosphatase and bilirubin. There may be leukocytosis in the presence of cholangitis, and coagulopathy.

Imaging. Transabdominal ultrasound, endoscopic retrograde cholangiopancreatography (ERCP) or MRCP may be useful in demonstrating the ductal dilations of the intrahepatic biliary system.

Liver biopsy may be needed in some cases to demonstrate the presence of congenital hepatic fibrosis.

Treatment. Antibiotics, often prolonged courses, are required for cholangitis. Intrahepatic stones may be difficult to remove by ERCP. Extracorporeal shock wave lithotripsy or intraductal electrohydraulic lithotripsy may be needed to clear intrahepatic stones, and cholangioscopic removal may be successful in some patients. Dissolution therapy using ursodeoxycholic acid for a long period (approximately 2 years) may be a useful adjunct.

Partial hepatectomy may be performed in patients with disease limited to one lobe. Patients who develop end-stage portal hypertension may require liver transplantation.

Oriental cholangiohepatitis

Etiology and pathogenesis. Oriental cholangiohepatitis, also called recurrent pyogenic cholangitis, is a disease of the biliary tree with multiple pigmented stones, biliary strictures and multiple bouts of cholangitis. Biliary parasites are implicated in the etiology of Oriental cholangiohepatitis. Liver flukes (*Clonorchis sinensis, Opisthorchis felineus, O. viverrini, Fasciola hepatica, F. giganta*) and roundworms (*Ascaris lumbricoides*) are the parasites most commonly involved in this disease. Bacterial infection and stasis further contribute to stone formation, stricturing and infection.

The pathogenesis of Oriental cholangiohepatitis is incompletely understood. The formation of multiple pigmented stones in the intrahepatic bile ducts proximal to biliary strictures results in recurrent cholangitis. Strictures may also affect the extrahepatic biliary system. The left hepatic system is more commonly involved, but the reasons for this are unclear.

Epidemiology and risk factors. Oriental cholangiohepatitis occurs in Far Eastern countries and in immigrants from the Far East to the West. Prevalence peaks in the third and fourth decades and is similar in men and women. The disease is more common in individuals with low socioeconomic status living in rural Asian communities.

Diagnosis

Symptoms and signs. Recurrent cholangitis occurs in 44% of patients, abdominal pain in 32% and pancreatitis (due to passage of a common bile duct stone) in 17%. Liver abscess, cirrhosis and rupture of biliary ducts, with fistula formation, may also occur.

Transabdominal ultrasonography may reveal bile duct dilation and stones. This is a useful initial test when the disease is clinically suspected.

Computed tomography may show dilated ducts, abscesses, stones or bilomas and may also be useful in mapping the extent of the disease.

Cholangiography. An MRCP scan can provide detailed visualization of the biliary system non-invasively but no therapy is possible, whereas ERCP, although more invasive, allows therapeutic intervention. In difficult cases percutaneous transhepatic cholangiography may be required to define the ductal system and intervene therapeutically.

Treatment. Biliary drainage is more difficult in Oriental cholangiohepatitis than with other causes of biliary obstruction and may be achieved using endoscopic, radiological or surgical methods, depending on local expertise. Treatment of acute cholangitis requires biliary drainage and antibiotics.

Cholangioscopy may be performed during ERCP or percutaneously and may allow lithotripsy and dilation of strictures. Stones recur in 30% of patients.

Surgery may involve cholecystectomy with common bile duct exploration; in a minority of patients (usually those with left hepatic disease), partial hepatic resection may be feasible.

Hepatic failure may occur due to cirrhosis. The risk of cholangiocarcinoma is 3–5%.

AIDS cholangiopathy

Etiology and pathogenesis. AIDS cholangiopathy is a disease syndrome in patients with AIDS that is characterized by biliary obstruction due to strictures caused by opportunistic infections. The organism most commonly implicated in AIDS cholangiopathy is *Cryptosporidium parvum*; microsporidia and *Cytomegalovirus* have also been implicated.

Epidemiology and risk factors. Before the advent of highly active antiretroviral therapy, the prevalence of cholangiopathy in patients with AIDS was about 25%. It usually occurs when the CD4 count is less than 100 cells/mm^3.

Diagnosis

Symptoms and signs. The most common symptoms and signs include right upper quadrant pain and diarrhea; jaundice and fever also occur. Liver function tests reveal the cholestatic picture, which may be normal in some patients.

Transabdominal ultrasonography is the initial screening procedure; if abnormal, further testing may be done to confirm the diagnosis.

Magnetic resonance cholangiopancreatography has not been widely evaluated in patients with AIDS cholangiopathy, but may be useful as a diagnostic test.

Endoscopic retrograde cholangiopancreatography allows the diagnosis to be confirmed and any indicated therapy performed. The most common findings on ERCP are sclerosing cholangitis and papillary stenosis (approximately 60%). Less commonly, either of these conditions may be found in isolation.

Medical treatment for infection (if the causative agent is identified) does not usually affect progression of this disease. In addition, AIDS cholangiopathy usually occurs in patients with advanced AIDS, and as such their survival is not likely to be determined by this condition. Ursodeoxycholic acid may help a small percentage of patients.

Endoscopic treatment. Sphincterotomy may be performed in patients with papillary stenosis and abdominal pain or jaundice. It provides pain relief for 23–70% of patients, but does not change strictures in the biliary tree. It is not helpful in the absence of papillary stenosis.

Primary sclerosing cholangitis

Etiology and pathogenesis. In primary sclerosing cholangitis (PSC), fibrotic strictures occur in the intra- and extrahepatic biliary system with no obvious cause. Genetic and immunologic factors are important in the pathogenesis of PSC. Up to 70% of patients with PSC may also have ulcerative colitis. Patients with PSC have an increased risk for cholangiocarcinoma, estimated at 1% per year. Biliary obstruction may cause secondary biliary cirrhosis and hepatic failure. The natural history of PSC is variable.

Epidemiology and risk factors. The mean age of presentation is between 40 and 50 years and the disease is more common in men than women. The presence of ulcerative colitis is the most important risk factor.

Diagnosis

Symptoms and signs include pruritus, jaundice, fatigue and abnormal liver function tests. Patients may present with symptoms and signs of end-stage liver disease and portal hypertension.

Magnetic resonance cholangiopancreatography should be used as a non-invasive method to image the biliary tree.

Endoscopic retrograde cholangiopancreatography. The diagnosis of PSC by ERCP also allows brushing and biopsy when cholangiocarcinoma is suspected.

Liver biopsy may be required in selected patients to assess the degree of liver fibrosis or to document the presence of cirrhosis in order to select appropriate therapy.

Treatment. Surgical resection may be an option in patients with significant hepatic fibrosis without cirrhosis; it may involve resection of the extrahepatic biliary tree and hepaticojejunostomy. Liver transplantation is the treatment of choice for patients with PSC and end-stage liver disease.

Prognosis. Median survival from the time of diagnosis is about 12 years. In patients without cirrhosis, 5-year survival is longer with surgical treatment (approximately 80%) than with non-surgical endoscopic treatment with sphincterotomy and balloon dilation of strictures (approximately 40%). Liver transplantation has a 5-year survival rate of more than 80%.

Future trends

- Molecular markers to improve diagnosis of cholangiocarcinoma in PSC.
- More trials with newer drugs.
- Improved preoperative assessment of resectability.
- Personalized targeted treatment based on genetic markers.

Key points – unusual diseases of the biliary tree

- More than 70% of patients with choledochal cysts have an abnormal pancreaticobiliary junction.
- Caroli's disease is a congenital condition resulting in multiple segmental dilations of intrahepatic ducts.
- Liver flukes and roundworms may cause Oriental cholangiohepatitis.
- AIDS cholangiopathy may result in right upper quadrant abdominal pain, biliary strictures and papillary stenosis.
- Up to 70% of patients with primary sclerosing cholangitis (PSC) may have ulcerative colitis.
- Liver transplantation is the treatment of choice for PSC with end-stage liver disease.

Key references

Ahrendt SA, Pitt HA, Kalloo AN et al. Primary sclerosing cholangitis: Resect, dilate or transplant? *Ann Surg* 1998;227:412–23.

Cello JP, Chan MF. Long-term follow-up of endoscopic retrograde cholangiopancreatography sphincterotomy for patients with acquired immune deficiency syndrome papillary stenosis. *Am J Med* 1995;99:600–3.

Chijiiwa K, Koga A. Surgical management and long-term follow-up of patients with choledochal cysts. *Am J Surg* 1993;165:238–42.

Eksteen B. Advances and controversies in the pathogenesis and management of primary sclerosing cholangitis. *Br Med Bull* 2014;110:89–98.

Lipsett PA, Pitt HA, Colombani PM et al. Choledochal cyst disease. A changing pattern of presentation. *Ann Surg* 1994;220:644–52.

Sherlock S. Overview of chronic cholestatic conditions in adults: terminology and definitions. *Clin Liver Dis* 1998;2:217–33.

Summerfield JA, Nagafuchi Y, Sherlock S et al. Hepatobiliary fibropolycystic diseases. A clinical and histological review of 51 patients. *J Hepatol* 1986;2:141–56.

Taylor AC, Palmer KR. Caroli's disease. *Eur J Gastroenterol Hepatol* 1998;10:105–8.

Todani T, Watanabe Y, Narusue M et al. Congenital bile duct cysts: classification, operative procedures, and review of thirty-seven cases including cancer arising from choledochal cyst. *Am J Surg* 1977;134:263–9.

Dysfunction of the sphincter of Oddi complex and gallbladder

Sphincter of Oddi dysfunction

Etiology and pathogenesis. The sphincter of Oddi is a complex of circular and longitudinal muscle fibers that surrounds the biliary and pancreatic sphincters where they open into the duodenum (Figure 7.1). Disorders of the sphincter of Oddi may present as sphincter stenosis or dyskinesia. Sphincter of Oddi stenosis is an actual anatomic narrowing of the sphincter, caused by inflammation, pancreatitis, gallstone passage or other unusual causes. Sphincter dyskinesia on the other hand is a spastic functional disorder of the sphincter, the cause of which is poorly understood.

Epidemiology and risk factors. Dysfunction mostly occurs after cholecystectomy, but it may occur in a patient with an intact gallbladder; this occurs more often in young women.

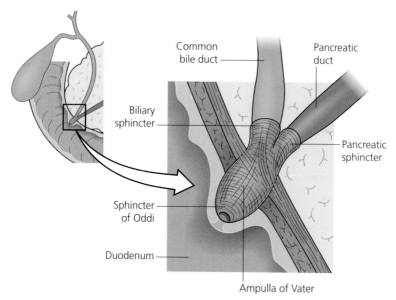

Figure 7.1 The sphincter of Oddi.

Diagnosis. The classification of the disorders of the biliary and pancreatic sphincters is described in Table 7.1.

Symptoms and signs include biliary-type pain and, in some patients, sphincter of Oddi dysfunction may present as recurrent pancreatitis. Pain is usually in the epigastrium or the right upper quadrant and may radiate to the back; it may also be associated with nausea and/or vomiting.

Cross-sectional imaging. Dilation of the common bile duct is seen on transabdominal ultrasound or endoscopic ultrasonography (EUS). Endoscopic retrograde cholangiopancreatography (ERCP) reveals dilation of the bile or pancreatic duct when drainage of contrast medium from the biliary or pancreatic ductal systems is delayed.

TABLE 7.1

Classification of biliary and pancreatic sphincter dysfunction

Features of biliary sphincter dysfunction

A   AST and ALT abnormal on at least two occasions and associated with abdominal pain

B   Dilated common bile duct on imaging

C   Delayed biliary drainage of contrast after ERCP or PTC

Features of pancreatic sphincter dysfunction

A   Abdominal pain with increased pancreatic enzymes (> 1.5 times normal)

B   Dilated pancreatic duct on imaging

C   Delayed pancreatic duct drainage of contrast after ERCP

Classification

- Type I dysfunction is associated with all three features (A, B and C)

- Type II dysfunction is associated with one or two features

- Type III dysfunction has none of the features

ALT, alanine aminotransferase; AST, aspartate aminotransferase; ERCP, endoscopic retrograde cholangiopancreatography; PTC, percutaneous transhepatic cholangiography.

Sphincter of Oddi manometry is the diagnostic gold standard. The biliary and pancreatic duct pressures are measured; an elevated basal pressure above 40 mmHg is diagnostic. A decrease in basal pressure after administration of a smooth muscle relaxant may help to differentiate between stenosis and spasm. Sphincter of Oddi manometry could be considered to confirm a diagnosis of type II biliary dysfunction. The limitations of this test include its invasiveness, lack of availability and an increased risk of pancreatitis (up to 20–30% in some series).

Provocation tests. An increase in the size of the bile duct (> 2 mm) after injection of cholecystokinin, or an increase in the size of the pancreatic duct (> 1.5 mm) after injection of secretin supports the diagnosis of biliary or pancreatic sphincter dysfunction, respectively.

Hepatobiliary scintigraphy with technetium-99m may help establish the existence of delayed biliary drainage and support a diagnosis of biliary sphincter dysfunction.

Medical treatment. A trial of smooth muscle relaxants may be useful, but results vary, and benefit may not be sustained in the long term or may be limited by side effects. Calcium channel blockers (nifedipine) and nitrates have also been tried. Oral nifedipine has been found to relieve pain in patients who had previously undergone cholecystectomy, and who had elevated basal pressure and sphincter of Oddi phasic contractions of predominantly antegrade nature.

Endoscopic treatment for all types of sphincter of Oddi dysfunction takes the form of biliary or pancreatic sphincterotomy during ERCP. Patients with type I biliary sphincter dysfunction respond well to sphincterotomy, which can be performed without manometry of the biliary sphincter. Type III biliary dysfunction is the hardest to treat, and there is no clear consensus on or understanding of invasive diagnostic procedures, treatment with sphincterotomy or the existence of other contributing or alternative causes of pain.

Pancreatic sphincterotomy may be undertaken if recurrent pancreatitis is considered to be related to pancreatic sphincter hypertension. Underlying chronic pancreatitis may adversely affect the outcome of pancreatic sphincterotomy via surgical or endoscopic methods.

A randomized sham-controlled trial of sphincterotomy in patients with pain after cholecystectomy, without significant imaging findings (dilated bile duct) or laboratory abnormalities, showed that sphincterotomy was not more effective than a sham procedure. Manometeric pressure abnormalities were not associated with the sphincterotomy outcome. This study mostly involved patients in the type III sphincter of Oddi dysfunction group. Based on this evidence-based study, some have suggested that sphincter of Oddi dysfunction type III is not a real disease and one should not pursue manometry or ERCP in these patients.

Gallbladder dyskinesia

Etiology and pathogenesis. Gallbladder dyskinesia is a disorder caused by abnormal motility or contraction of the gallbladder in the absence of gallstones. Surgical resection of a dysfunctional dyskinetic gallbladder reveals acalculous chronic cholecystitis in some patients. The pathogenesis is unclear but it is regarded as a motility disorder as patients frequently have other gastrointestinal motility disorders. Functional gallbladder disorder is a relatively new term used by some to describe gallbladder dyskinesia.

Epidemiology and risk factors. The exact frequency of gallbladder dyskinesia is unknown. This is a diagnosis of exclusion. Patients with other gastrointestinal motility disorders are likely to be at increased risk.

Diagnosis. Liver function tests and white cell count are normal. Transabdominal ultrasonography shows a normal-sized common bile duct and no stones in the gallbladder. Other investigations (e.g. endoscopy, EUS and CT) may be needed to rule out other causes of right upper quadrant pain.

Symptoms and signs include intermittent right upper quadrant pain, often postprandially. Nausea and vomiting also occur, possibly related to intake of fatty food.

Cholecystokinin-stimulated scintigraphy. A ^{99}Tc–HIDA (technetium-labeled hepatobiliary iminodiacetic acid) scan with gallbladder stimulation by intravenous administration of cholecystokinin (CCK) can be used to calculate the gallbladder ejection fraction. An ejection fraction below 35–40% is considered abnormal and these patients are more likely to respond to cholecystectomy. In some patients the pain of gallbladder dyskinesia is reproduced when CCK is administered.

Treatment is by cholecystectomy, usually laparoscopic. In patients whose gallbladder ejection fraction by CCK-stimulated scintigraphy is less than 35–40%, a significant number will experience improvement or resolution of pain following cholecystectomy.

Before attempting cholecystectomy other diagnoses need to be eliminated as a cause for the patient's abdominal pain. Careful selection of appropriate patients for cholecystectomy must be undertaken. Treatment by cholecystectomy for this condition is controversial.

Key points – dysfunction of the sphincter of Oddi complex and gallbladder

- Sphincter of Oddi dysfunction may be due to anatomic stenosis or a spastic functional disorder, and is most common after cholecystectomy. A lot of controversy surrounds this topic.
- Data suggest that sphincterotomy is not more effective than a sham procedure in patients with type III dysfunction, leading some to suggest type III dysfunction may not be a real disease.
- Sphincter of Oddi manometry is the diagnostic gold standard for the dysfunction. Biliary or pancreatic duct pressure of more than 40 mmHg is diagnostic of biliary or pancreatic sphincter dysfunction, respectively.
- A low gallbladder ejection fraction of less than 35–40% on ^{99}Tc–HIDA (hepatobiliary iminodiacetic acid) scan with gallbladder stimulation may be diagnostic of gallbladder dyskinesia (functional gallbladder disorder), and is the best predictor of response to cholecystectomy.
- The pain of gallbladder dyskinesia is reproduced in some patients when cholecystokinin is administered.

Future trends

- Improved understanding of the pathophysiology and pain-causing mechanisms attributed to sphincter of Oddi dysfunction so far.
- Improved understanding of other diseases and mechanisms that cause pain similar to, or overlapping with, pain considered to be from sphincter of Oddi dysfunction and gallbladder dyskinesia/ functional gallbladder disorder.

Key references

Baillie J, Kimberly J. Prospective comparison of secretin-stimulated MRCP with manometry in the diagnosis of sphincter of Oddi dysfunction types II and III. *Gut* 2007;56:742–4.

Chuttani R, Carr-Locke DL. Pathophysiology of the sphincter of Oddi. *Surg Clin North Am* 1993;73:1311–22.

Cotton PB, Durkalski V, Romagnuolo J et al. Effect of endoscopic sphincterotomy for suspected sphincter of Oddi dysfunction on pain-related disability following cholecystectomy: the EPISOD randomized clinical trial. *JAMA* 2014;311:2101–9.

Dawwas MF, Bruno MJ, Lee JG. Endoscopic sphincterotomy for sphincter of Oddi dysfunction: inefficacious therapy for a fictitious disease. *Gastroenterology* 2015;148:440–3.

Gurusamy KS, Junnarkar S, Farouk M, Davidson BR. Cholecystectomy for suspected gallbladder dyskinesia. *Cochrane Database Syst Rev* 2009;1:CD007086.

Leung WD, Sherman S. Endoscopic approach to the patient with motility disorders of the bile duct and sphincter of Oddi. *Gastrointest Endosc Clin N Am* 2013;23:405–34.

Neoptolemos JP, Bailey IS, Carr-Locke DL. Sphincter of Oddi dysfunction: results of treatment by endoscopic sphincterotomy. *Br J Surg* 1988;75:454–9.

Pfau PR, Banerjee S, Barth BA et al. Sphincter of Oddi manometry. *Gastrointest Endosc* 2011;74: 1175–80.

Sgouros SN, Pereira SP. Systematic review: sphincter of Oddi dysfunction--non-invasive diagnostic methods and long-term outcome after endoscopic sphincterotomy. *Aliment Pharmacol Ther* 2006;24:237–46.

Stinton LM, Shaffer EA. Epidemiology of gallbladder disease: cholelithiasis and cancer. *Gut Liver* 2012;6:172–87.

Etiology and pathogenesis

Most cases of acute pancreatitis can be explained by gallstones, alcohol consumption or idiopathic pancreatitis (Figure 8.1), although there are many other causes (Table 8.1).

Under normal physiological circumstances, pancreatic enzymes are released in a non-activated form (principally as proenzymes) into the pancreatic ductules from secretory granules in pancreatic acini. Secretion is stimulated either by cholecystokinin (also known as pancreozymin) released from the duodenum upon entry of food, or by acetylcholine following neural stimulation. Normally, trypsinogen is activated to trypsin in the duodenal lumen by the action of enterokinase. Once activated, trypsin in turn activates all the other proenzymes in the pancreatic juice in the duodenal lumen. Trypsin also activates itself, resulting in exponential amplification of trypsin activity.

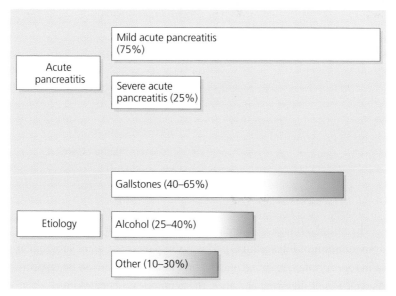

Figure 8.1 Etiology of acute pancreatitis.

71

TABLE 8.1

Causes of acute pancreatitis

Common causes	Less common causes
• Gallstones	• Viral infection (mumps, human immunodeficiency virus)
• Alcohol consumption	
• Idiopathic pancreatitis	• *Ascaris lumbricoides* (endemic areas)
• Endoscopic retrograde cholangiopancreatography	• Scorpion bite (Trinidad and other endemic areas)
• External trauma	• Closed-loop duodenal obstruction
• Intraoperative trauma	
• Pancreatic cancer	• Pancreatic stricture (postirradiation)
• Ampullary cancer	
• Pancreatic surgery	• Anti-acetylcholinesterase-containing insecticides
• Ischemia	• Cobra venom
• Postoperative (cardiac, renal and urological surgery)	• Periampullary duodenal wall cysts
• Hyperlipidemia	• Hypercalcemia – hyperparathyroidism
• Hypothermia	• Steroids
	• Annular pancreas
	• Hereditary pancreatitis
	• Isolated autoimmune chronic pancreatitis
	• Pancreatic divisum
	• Sphincter of Oddi disorders (see Chapter 7)

The initial damage of acute pancreatitis begins with the dysregulation of intracellular pathways in pancreatic acini subsequent to inappropriate trypsinogen activation and autodigestion by trypsin. As well as self-digesting enzymes, the acini release chemokines, promoting an extensive inflammatory cell infiltrate.

There are several theories for the pathogenesis of acute pancreatitis, all of which are controversial. One considers Ca^{2+} homeostasis. It is thought that disruption of homeostasis leads to severe depletion of Ca^{2+} stores and cytosolic Ca^{2+} overload, triggering either apoptosis or necrosis of pancreatic acinar cells. Other theories include:

- gallstone migration
- common bile–pancreatic duct
- excessive leukocyte activation
- microcirculation disturbance theory.

The disease quickly resolves in 75% of patients, but in the other 25% the attack is severe. Excessive stimulation of white blood cells, coupled with the release of acute-phase proteins from the liver results in systemic inflammatory response syndrome (SIRS) (Figure 8.2).

Unlike chronic pancreatitis, once the patient has recovered from an attack of acute pancreatitis there may be complete resolution of

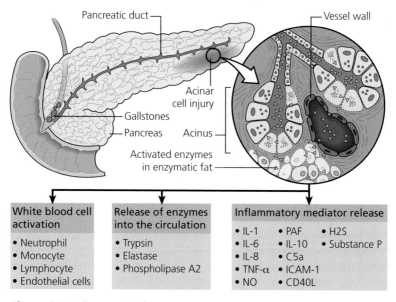

Figure 8.2 Pathogenesis of acute pancreatitis. Apoptosis or necrosis of pancreatic acinar cells leads to a systemic inflammatory response syndrome, with white blood cell activity and the release of enzymes and inflammatory mediators. C5a, complement 5a; H2S, hydrogen sulphide; IL, interleukin; NO, nitric oxide; PAF, platelet-activating factor; TNF, tumor necrosis factor.

symptoms and a return to normal anatomy and physiology. However, further attacks are likely if the initiating cause has not been removed (gallstones, alcohol consumption, etc.) or there has been major pancreatic necrosis, resulting in chronic pancreatitis or main pancreatic duct stricture.

Epidemiology and risk factors

The incidence of acute pancreatitis varies from 20 to 120 per 100 000 in the general population and is increasing steadily as a result of an aging population and increasing alcohol consumption.

Diagnosis

Symptoms and signs. Acute pancreatitis is divided into interstitial edematous pancreatitis and necrotizing pancreatitis; they both have a similar initial presentation. A sudden and severe onset of epigastric pain may remain in the epigastrium or spread into the central back and the whole of the abdomen. The patient may be unable to move because of the pain, refuse food and water, and may vomit. These symptoms are accompanied by SIRS, which comprises two or more of:

- core temperature above 38°C or below 36°C
- heart rate above 90 beats/minute
- respiratory rate greater than 20 breaths/minute or $PaCO_2$ below 4.3 kPa (32 mmHg)
- white cell count above 12×10^9 cells/L, below 4×10^9 cells/L, or more than 10% immature cells.

Common symptoms and signs (Table 8.2) may be confused with those of a number of acute conditions above or below the diaphragm:

- perforated peptic ulcer
- leaking aortic aneurysm
- mesenteric infarction
- myocardial infarction
- perforated esophagus
- gastroesophageal reflux
- pneumonia
- acute cholecystitis or biliary colic
- peptic ulcer disease.

TABLE 8.2

Symptoms and signs of acute pancreatitis

Common findings	Less common findings
• Abdominal pain	• Ascites
• Nausea and vomiting	• Symptomatic hypocalcemia
• Abdominal tenderness	• Massive intra-abdominal hemorrhage
• Paralytic ileus	• Disseminated intravascular coagulation
• Fever	
• Abdominal distension	• Subcutaneous fat necrosis
• Tachycardia	• Hepatic portal vein thrombosis
• Tachypnea	• Periumbilical darkening of the skin (from blood) – Cullen's sign
• Jaundice	
• Respiratory insufficiency	• Local areas of discoloration in the region of the loins (due to retroperitoneal hemorrhage) – Grey Turner's sign
• Hypovolemia	
• Shock	
• Pleural effusion	• Infra-inguinal bruising – Fox's sign
• Cardiac insufficiency	
• Renal insufficiency	• Pericardial effusion
	• Cardiac tamponade
	• Hematemesis
	• Melena
	• Polyarthritis
	• Bone marrow fat necrosis
	• Focal cerebral necrosis
	• Encephalopathy
	• Sudden blindness

Laboratory tests. The diagnosis is based on a typical clinical presentation (abdominal pain with acute onset of persistent severe epigastric pain radiating to the back), plus a serum lipase (or amylase) that is three times the normal upper limit within 2–3 days of the onset of symptoms. The serum amylase peaks at about 24 hours after the onset of the attack and then declines exponentially over the next 5–7 days. Thus, if the amylase is measured at day 4 or 5 after the onset of the attack, it may be only marginally raised or within normal limits. Urinary amylase may be cleared more slowly, but the diagnostic threshold is much higher (tenfold). An elevated serum alanine transaminase level (> 60 IU/L) within 48 hours of an attack is highly indicative of a possible biliary cause.

Imaging. Absence of gas on an erect plain abdominal and chest radiograph will eliminate most large gastrointestinal perforations. The presence of gallbladder stones is often missed by abdominal ultrasound during an acute attack, but endoscopic ultrasonography (EUS) has high sensitivity and specificity for the diagnosis of gallstones, especially small stones (< 3 mm; microlithiasis). MRI or transabdominal ultrasound are used less commonly for the initial diagnosis.

> If there is any doubt about the diagnosis, an emergency CT scan must be performed.

The majority of patients have diffuse enlargement of the pancreas due to edema, with symptoms that usually resolve rapidly. Up to 10% of patients have necrosis of the pancreatic and peripancreatic tissues, which continues for several days, with variable evolution towards persistence or disappearance, remaining sterile or becoming infected.

Based on the revised Atlanta classification, the presence of fluid alone and the presence of necrosis with variable amounts of fluid about the pancreas are important distinctions in the definition of acute pancreatitis type.

Treatment

Predicting severity. It is important to determine as early as possible (within the first 3 days of symptom onset) whether the attack of pancreatitis is likely to be mild or severe:

- acute pancreatitis (includes mild acute pancreatitis; no organ failure, no local or systemic complications)
- moderately severe acute pancreatitis (transient organ failure, local or systemic complications without persistent organ failure)
- severe acute pancreatitis (persistent organ failure over 48 hours).

Clinical judgment can be difficult, especially during the first 24–48 hours when the severity of disease may change rapidly. One or more of the following methods may be used.

Computed tomography scanning is used to help establish the diagnosis in uncertain cases and to assist in determining the need for and extent of surgical intervention (pancreatic necrosectomy, colectomy for necrosis, etc.).

Pancreatitis severity is usually stratified into mild, moderate and severe, based on the extent of inflammatory changes, fluid collections and necrosis seen in CT scans.

Balthazar score. The original Balthazar score referred only to the grading of pancreatitis (based on pancreas enlargement and number of fluid collections). It was modified into the CT severity index by including grading of necrosis extent. The maximum score is 10 – the sum of the scores for the grading of pancreatitis and necrosis (Table 8.3).

Serum C-reactive protein (CRP) above 150 mg/L indicates a severe attack, but the peak is not reached until 72 hours after symptom onset.

Clinicobiochemical criteria. The Ranson score includes 11 criteria variously applicable at 24 and 48 hours, and separate systems for alcohol- and gallstone-associated acute pancreatitis. The Imrie or Glasgow system is much simpler, requiring only eight criteria at 48 hours, and is just as accurate (Table 8.4).

APACHE II score (Acute Physiology and Chronic Health Evaluation) can be applied at any time but is cumbersome, requiring 15 different clinical and biochemical criteria.

Medical treatment. The principles are basic resuscitation and close monitoring in an appropriate setting, ranging from an acute admissions ward to an intensive therapy unit.

TABLE 8.3

The CT severity index

Grading of pancreatitis

- A: normal pancreas (0)
- B: pancreas enlargement (1)
- C: inflammatory changes in the pancreas and peripancreatic fat (2)
- D: ill-defined single fluid collections (3)
- E: ≥ 2 poorly defined fluid collections (4)

Grading of pancreatic necrosis

- None (0)
- < 30% (2)
- 30–50% (4)
- > 50% (6)

CT, computed tomography.

TABLE 8.4

Glasgow or Imrie criteria for predicting the severity of an attack of acute pancreatitis

The mnemonic 'PANCREAS' makes this easy to remember.

P   Arterial PaO_2 < 9 kPa

A   Albumin < 32 g/L

N   Urea nitrogen > 10 mmol/L

C   Calcium < 2 mmol/L

R   Raised white cell count: > 16 mmol/L

E   Enzyme: lactate dehydrogenase > 600 mmol/L

A   Age > 55 years

S   Sugar: glucose >10 mmol/L

The presence of ≥ 3 criteria reached before or at 48 hours of an attack predicts a severe attack; ≤ 2 criteria predicts a mild attack. The maximum sensitivity for a severe attack and the maximum specificity for a mild attack are achieved at 48 hours after the start of an attack.

The essential requirements are as follows:
- 1–4 hourly monitoring of pulse, blood pressure, temperature and urine output
- baseline chest radiograph and measurement of arterial blood gases
- complete blood count (including thrombocytes) and measurement of basic electrolytes, albumin, proteins, liver enzymes, bilirubin, calcium, glucose, urea, creatinine and CRP.

Overviews of the management for mild and severe attacks are given in Figures 8.3 and 8.4, respectively.

Mild acute pancreatitis. Patients require fasting and fluid replacement to counteract hypovolemia and hypotension until disappearance of pain and normalization of amylase/lipase. Nasogastric aspiration might be needed if vomiting is persistent.

Severe acute pancreatitis. Patients with a severe attack have persistent organ failure (over 48 hours from onset) and will need to be managed on an intensive care unit. Treatment is usually supportive with vigorous fluid resuscitation, reaching 6–8 liters per day (at least 250–500 mL per hour of isotonic crystalloid solution) in severe cases. Fluid loading (rapid fluid perfusions) or volume expansion is imperative in the clinical management, allowing fast correction of hypovolemia and cardiac/circulatory dysfunction. Patients may also require two or more of the following:
- continuous arterial and central venous pressure monitoring
- intubation for assisted respiratory ventilation
- inotropes for cardiac support
- hemofiltration or hemodialysis for renal failure
- nutrition by a nasojejunal tube to provide early enteral nutrition.

Compared to parenteral feeding, enteral feeding reduces infectious complications, surgical interventions and mortality in acute pancreatitis. However, additional parenteral nutrition may be required for sufficient calories.

Pain management requires meperidine (50–100 mg every 4–6 hours) for patients without renal failure. High glucose levels (over 200 mg/dL or 11.1 mmol/L) should be managed with insulin. Antisecretory agents (glucagon, somatostatin or octreotide) have not proven beneficial.

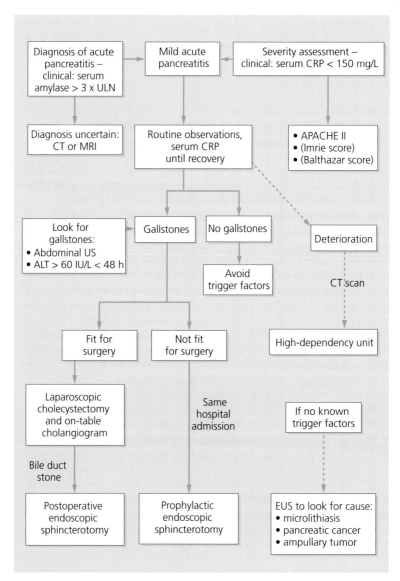

Figure 8.3 Management of mild acute pancreatitis. ALT, alanine aminotransferase; APACHE, Acute Physiology And Chronic Health Evaluation; CRP, C-reactive protein; CT, computed tomography; EUS, endoscopic ultrasonography; ULN, upper limit of normal; US, ultrasonography.

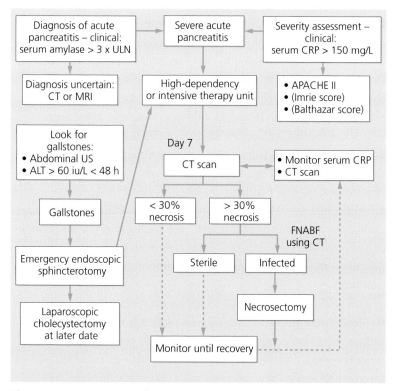

Figure 8.4 Management of severe acute pancreatitis. ALT, alanine aminotransferase; APACHE, Acute Physiology And Chronic Health Evaluation; CRP, C-reactive protein; CT, computed tomography; FNABF, fine needle aspiration for bacteriology and fungi; ULN, upper limit of normal; US, ultrasonography.

Protease inhibitors and anti-inflammatory/antioxidant agents need further clinical studies.

Antibiotics are routinely used for extrapancreatic infections (cholangitis, sepsis, pneumonia, etc.) but are not recommended for prophylactic use in severe acute pancreatitis, even in the presence of sterile necrosis. However, if infected necrosis is suspected (based on failure to improve) or documented (by CT-guided fine needle aspiration), then antibiotics are recommended, followed by necrosectomy if required.

Endoscopic treatment. Urgent endoscopic retrograde cholangiopancreatography (ERCP), undertaken less than 24 hours from onset with an intention to complete endoscopic sphincterotomy, should be performed in patients with acute pancreatitis and concurrent acute cholangitis due to retained common bile duct (CBD) stones. ERCP is usually not indicated in mild or moderately severe acute biliary pancreatitis without cholangitis or CBD obstruction. However, in patients with predicted severe acute pancreatitis secondary to gallstones, when imaging and biochemical tests highly predict an obstructed CBD (even without cholangitis), ERCP will possibly reduce morbidity and mortality from acute pancreatitis. EUS and magnetic resonance cholangiopancreatography are needed to prove the presence of suspected CBD stones, and will prevent unnecessary ERCP in patients with acute biliary pancreatitis without cholangitis and/or jaundice.

EUS-guided drainage is a good option for symptomatic pancreatic fluid collections (especially for pseudocysts). It is less invasive than surgery, has fewer complications (compared to percutaneous and surgical options), a lower mortality rate and high technical and clinical success. EUS-guided necrosectomy is an option for suspected or confirmed infected necrosis, especially walled-off necrosis. Thus, if possible, interventions should be postponed for at least 4 weeks to allow the collections to be walled-off.

A cholecystectomy should be performed in all patients with acute biliary pancreatitis, as they run a high risk of recurrent attacks of acute pancreatitis, along with the attendant morbidity and mortality.

Surgical treatment may be required in necrotizing acute pancreatitis if infected necrosis is present or suspected (based on clinical deterioration or prolonged organ failure). It should, however, be postponed as much as possible in favor of minimally invasive radiological or endoscopic drainage options.

The principal purpose of surgery in severe acute pancreatitis is the removal of necrotic pancreatic tissue (necrosectomy). Surgery is indicated (relatively) in extensive sterile pancreatic necrosis where there is no improvement of symptoms following at least 2 weeks of optimal care from the detection of extensive necrosis. Drainage is indicated in cases with symptoms of obstruction (gastrointestinal or biliary), although it should be postponed for at least 4 weeks to allow liquefaction of the contents and development of a fibrous wall (walled-off necrosis). Minimally invasive methods include percutaneous (CT or ultrasound guided) or endoscopic methods (EUS-guided drainage and necrosectomy), as well as minimally invasive retroperitoneal necrosectomy. Most tertiary referral centers prefer these methods to open necrosectomy.

Because the features of SIRS are identical to those of sepsis (defined as SIRS with proven infection), clinical parameters may not identify pancreatic infection before it is too late. Thus, from day 7 of a severe attack, all patients must undergo a contrast-enhanced CT scan, repeated at 7–10-day intervals until there are signs of clinical improvement. Three main techniques can be used for necrosectomy:

- open necrosectomy with closed lesser sac lavage
- repeated laparotomies with zipper to close the peritoneum after each intervention or left open as laparostomy
- minimally invasive necrosectomy – EUS-guided transgastric necrosectomy or videoscopic retroperitoneal approach have the best results.

Complications

SIRS is a feature of the first phase of acute pancreatitis, and as such is not regarded as a complication but as a manifestation of the disease. However, a severe SIRS response will promote systemic complications that lead to multi-organ dysfunction syndrome (MODS).

Local complications. The revised Atlanta classification includes peripancreatic fluid collection, pancreatic pseudocyst, pancreatic and peripancreatic necrosis and walled-off necrosis as local complications. Other local complications include infections, portal/splenic vein thrombosis, hemorrhage, colonic necrosis and pancreatic fistulas.

Acute peripancreatic fluid collections are common in acute pancreatitis, even in mild acute pancreatitis. They are not lined by either granulation (inflammatory) or fibrous tissue. The natural history

83

is usually one of spontaneous resolution. Acute fluid collections that are rich in pancreatic enzymes may progress to pancreatic pseudocysts.

Pancreatic pseudocysts are rich in pancreatic enzymes and encapsulated by granulation (inflammatory) and fibrous tissue (Figure 8.5). By definition, a pseudocyst will not be properly formed for at least 4 weeks from the start of an attack. Most pseudocysts resolve spontaneously, but when symptomatic and persistent (> 6 weeks) they should be drained, preferably by minimal invasive approaches (transluminal with endoscopic ultrasound guidance or transpapillary during ERCP).

Pancreatic necrosis is accurately determined by contrast-enhanced CT (Figure 8.6). It may be observed early during an attack but often develops progressively – necrosis of less than 30% is rarely of clinical significance. Initially the necrosis is not infected (sterile pancreatic necrosis); however, infection can develop and this is associated with increased morbidity and mortality.

Infected pancreatic necrosis is a secondary infection of sterile pancreatic necrosis and develops in the later phase in 40–70% of patients with severe disease. By definition it is retroperitoneal and commonly extends down the left and sometimes right paracolic gutter surrounding the kidneys. The necrosis may extend into the pelvis or chest and occurs through the spread of bacteria from the gastrointestinal

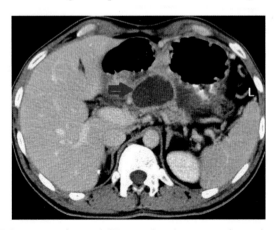

Figure 8.5 Contrast-enhanced CT scan showing a pseudocyst located at the level of the pancreatic body with a defined wall (capsule).

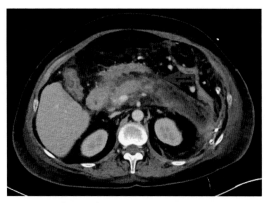

Figure 8.6 Contrast-enhanced CT scan in a patient with severe acute pancreatitis, showing pancreatic edema, as well as fluid and necrosis at the level of the pancreatic body and tail.

tract, biliary tree, skin or iatrogenic intervention. Gas-forming bacteria are commonly involved and gas within the area of infected pancreatic necrosis is a common late feature. The infected necrosis acts as a major focus of infection, leading to septicemia and amplification of SIRS and MODS. The overall mortality in this group of patients is 20–40%.

Secondary fungal infection is frequently associated with antibiotic treatment of infected pancreatic necrosis and significantly raises mortality.

Portal and/or splenic vein thrombosis is associated with protracted recovery from extensive pancreatic necrosis. The consequence is left-sided portal hypertension, with the development of venous collaterals and gastric varices.

Hemorrhage may occur from necrotizing pancreatitis and erosion of major vessels within or close to the pancreas.

Colonic necrosis may occur because of involvement of colonic vessels (commonly the middle colic and marginal arteries), leading to colonic necrosis and fecal peritonitis.

Pancreatic fistula. A fistula is usually an abnormal communication between two epithelial surfaces, but the term is also used if there is an abnormal communication between a hollow viscus, such as the colon or duodenum, and an area of pancreatic necrosis. This leads to gas within the area of pancreatic necrosis.

Systemic complications. The assessment of several organ systems should be included. Likely systemic complications of acute pancreatitis include the following.

- Respiratory failure, which may include unilateral or bilateral pleural effusions and may progress to full-blown adult respiratory distress syndrome.
- Cardiovascular failure with low systolic blood pressure (< 90 mmHg).
- Renal failure with increased serum creatinine (> 1.4 mg/dL; > 134 µmol/L).
- Central nervous system disturbances, including coma.
- Metabolic abnormalities, which may include low arterial pH, low serum calcium and albumin and raised blood glucose and urea.
- Coagulation disorders, which may include reduced clotting and abnormal platelet function, and may lead to disseminated intravascular coagulation with massive systemic bleeding.
- MODS, more than one system may fail in the early phase (the first 2 weeks) of a severe attack; in the later phases multi-organ failure is usually secondary to sepsis from infected pancreatic necrosis.

The latest definitions in the international consensus from 2012 state that persistent organ failure should be differentiated from systemic complications, which are exacerbations of pre-existing comorbidities.

Follow-up

In order to prevent further attacks, known triggers should be avoided (for example alcohol, if that was the cause). If there is no known trigger then EUS should be used to look for a cause – particularly microlithiasis (small gallstones), pancreatic cancer or ampullary tumors.

There are no long-term sequelae following recovery from mild acute pancreatitis. In severe necrotizing pancreatitis, however, there are significant late complications in up to 60% of patients. These include:

- delayed collections or pseudocysts
- pancreatic exocrine insufficiency
- diabetes mellitus
- biliary stricture.

Thus, long-term follow-up is required to monitor the development of these complications.

Key points – acute pancreatitis

- An urgent CT scan of the abdomen should be performed if there is any doubt about the diagnosis of acute pancreatitis.
- Prognostic evaluation for the severity of the disease should be completed within the first 3 days of symptom onset.
- It should be determined whether gallstones are the cause of the attack; if so, urgent endoscopic sphincterotomy should be performed in severe cases; all cases of acute biliary pancreatitis usually require cholecystectomy.
- If severe acute pancreatitis with extensive necrosis is found beyond the first week, fine needle aspiration for bacteriology and fungi should be performed; if there is proven infected necrosis, pancreatic necrosectomy might be required.
- If the etiology is uncertain, endoscopic ultrasonography should be performed following resolution of the attack to exclude unusual causes of obstruction such as small stones or tumors.

Future trends

- Early prognostication using one or two rapid blood tests.
- More extensive use of emergency endoscopic sphincterotomy for bile duct stones in severe disease.
- Improved and earlier detection of infected pancreatic necrosis.
- Better results from minimally invasive pancreatic necrosectomy.
- Drugs that will modify the progression of mild to severe acute pancreatitis.
- More effective measures to treat the excessive systemic inflammatory response syndrome and prevent multi-organ dysfunction.
- Better treatment of multi-organ failure.

Key references

Bakker OJ, Issa Y, van Santvoort HC et al. Treatment options for acute pancreatitis. *Nat Rev Gastroenterol Hepatol* 2014;11:462–9.

Banks PA, Bollen TL, Dervenis C et al. Classification of acute pancreatitis – 2012: revision of the Atlanta classification and definitions by international consensus. *Gut* 2013; 62:102–11.

Bortolotti P, Saulnier F, Colling D et al. New tools for optimizing fluid resuscitation in acute pancreatitis. *World J Gastroenterol* 2014;20:16113–22.

Fisher JM, Gardner TB. Endoscopic therapy of necrotizing pancreatitis and pseudocysts. *Gastrointest Endosc Clin N Am* 2013;23:787–802.

Frossard JL, Lescuyer P, Pastor CM. Experimental evidence of obesity as a risk factor for severe acute pancreatitis. *World J Gastroenterol* 2009;15:5260–5.

Kambhampati S, Park W, Habtezion A. Pharmacologic therapy for acute pancreatitis. *World J Gastroenterol* 2014;20:16868–80.

Oláh A, Romics L Jr. Enteral nutrition in acute pancreatitis: a review of the current evidence. *World J Gastroenterol* 2014;20:16123–31.

Ong JP, Fock KM. Nutritional support in acute pancreatitis. *J Dig Dis* 2012;13:445–52.

Seewald S, Ang TL, Richter H et al. Long-term results after endoscopic drainage and necrosectomy of symptomatic pancreatic fluid collections. *Dig Endosc* 2012;24:36–41.

Seifert H, Biermer M, Schmitt W et al. Transluminal endoscopic necrosectomy after acute pancreatitis: a multicentre study with long-term follow-up (the GEPARD Study). *Gut* 2009;58:1260–6.

Seta T, Noguchi Y, Shikata S, Nakayama T. Treatment of acute pancreatitis with protease inhibitors administered through intravenous infusion: an updated systematic review and meta-analysis. *BMC Gastroenterol* 2014;14:102.

Surlin V, Săftoiu A, Dumitrescu D. Imaging tests for accurate diagnosis of acute biliary pancreatitis. *World J Gastroenterol* 2014;20:16544–9.

Tenner S, Baillie J, DeWitt J et al. American College of Gastroenterology guideline: management of acute pancreatitis. *Am J Gastroenterol* 2013;108:1400–15.

Trikudanathan G, Attam R, Arain MA et al. Endoscopic interventions for necrotizing pancreatitis. *Am J Gastroenterol* 2014;109:969–81.

van Santvoort HC, Besselink MG, Bakker OJ et al. A step-up approach or open necrosectomy for necrotizing pancreatitis. *N Engl J Med* 2010;362:1491–502.

Working Group IAP/APA Acute Pancreatitis Guidelines. IAP/APA evidence-based guidelines for the management of acute pancreatitis. *Pancreatology* 2013;13(4 Suppl 2):e1-15.

Etiology and pathogenesis

Chronic pancreatitis is a progressive inflammatory process of the pancreas that leads to irreversible functional and morphological destruction of the pancreas. The pathological features of chronic pancreatitis are:

- disruption of the lobular parenchymal architecture, with extensive destruction of pancreatic acini (and subsequently islets of Langerhans) and replacement by fibrous or fatty tissue
- chronic inflammatory infiltrate
- pancreatic ductal and parenchymal calcification.

The pathogenesis of chronic pancreatitis varies slightly according to the etiology and, once initiated, the disease follows a relentless course. Several theories explain the pathogenesis of chronic pancreatitis, although none is perfect. The initial hypothesis suggested an increased concentration of ductal proteins that form plugs which later calcify. However, this has been challenged by the necrosis–fibrosis concept, which theorizes the disease is initiated by repeated bouts of pancreatitis due to the action of tumor growth factor (TGF)-α and TGF-β.

The primary injury appears to occur in the acinar cells, but injury to the pancreatic ducts may also be contributory. As a consequence of this injury, stellate cells are stimulated to produce excessive amounts of fibrous tissues (Figure 9.1). As the disease progresses, chronic inflammation not only destroys the gland itself but has major effects on surrounding structures, with serious consequences (Table 9.1).

Autoimmune pancreatitis (AIP) is a rare fibroinflammatory disorder of the pancreas with two described types: type 1 (associated with extrapancreatic manifestations and high levels of immunoglobulin [IgG] 4-positive cells) and type 2 (with a few IgG4-positive cells found predominantly in the pancreas). Although IgG4 autoantibodies are associated with AIP, the mechanisms are not completely clear. However, it is known that cell-mediated immunity (cytotoxic T cell responses), complement and molecular mimicry are involved.

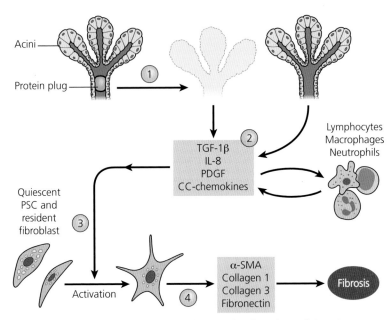

Figure 9.1 Schematic representation of the pathophysiology of chronic pancreatitis (CP). 1) A protein plug obstructs the acinar duct triggering acinar cell apoptosis and necrosis. 2) Necrotic and apoptotic cells and neighboring epithelial and mesenchymal cells release cytokines and chemokines, triggering an inflammatory infiltrate which also releases cytokines and chemokines. 3) Cytokines stimulate the differentiation of quiescent pancreatic stellate cells (PSCs) and resident fibroblasts into myofibroblast-like phenotypes. 4) Activated PSCs and myofibroblasts secrete α-smooth muscle actin (α-SMA) and fibrillar collagens resulting in the characteristic fibrosis seen in CP.

Epidemiology and risk factors

The prevalence of chronic pancreatitis varies enormously, from 20 to 200 per 100 000 in the general population, and is increasing as a result of environmental factors, in particular the rising consumption of alcohol and tobacco smoking, which are both regarded as independent risk factors. Approximately 70% of cases are associated with alcohol consumption, and approximately 25% of the remaining cases are classed as idiopathic. AIP is rare (< 1 per 100 000), with published case series from tertiary referral centers. The peak age of onset occurs after 60 years of age.

TABLE 9.1

Complications of chronic pancreatitis

- Pancreatic exocrine deficiency, leading to severe weight loss
- Pancreatic endocrine insufficiency, leading to diabetes mellitus and requiring insulin therapy
- Pain
- Pseudocyst
- Stricture of the main pancreatic duct
- Main pancreatic duct stones
- Parenchymal stones
- Biliary obstruction
- Duodenal obstruction
- Pancreatic ascites – free pancreatic juice in the abdominal cavity secondary to disruption of the main pancreatic duct or a communicating pseudocyst
- Pancreatic fistula – an abnormal communication between the main pancreatic duct and an internal organ (such as the peritoneal cavity) or the skin (external fistula)
- Left-sided portal hypertension – selective increased venous pressure in the left side of the hepatic portal system, causing gastric varices
- Pseudoaneurysm – commonly caused by erosion of a pseudocyst into a major visceral vessel (such as the splenic artery or celiac trunk)
- Pancreatic ductal adenocarcinoma (20-fold increased risk or 5% of all patients)
- Social and professional disruption

Additional factors that contribute to the development of chronic pancreatitis, and an individual's susceptibility to it, include genetic factors (see Chapter 10). Three genes, *CFTR, PRSS1, SPINK1* are recognized to be involved, and a high proportion of patients with idiopathic chronic pancreatitis have mutations in the *CFTR* and *SPINK1* genes (Table 9.2)

TABLE 9.2

Classification of chronic pancreatitis

Toxic–metabolic pancreatitis

- Alcohol consumption
- Tobacco smoking
- Hypocalcemia – hyperparathyroidism
- Chronic renal failure
- Medications
- Phenacetin abuse (possibly from chronic renal insufficiency)
- Toxins
- Organotin compounds (e.g. di-n-butyltin dichloride)

Idiopathic pancreatitis

- Early-onset
- Late onset
- Tropical
- Tropical calcific pancreatitis
- Fibrocalculous pancreatic diabetes

Hereditary pancreatitis

- Autosomal-dominant – mutations in the PRSS1 gene (also known as the cationic trypsinogen gene)
- Autosomal-recessive and modifier genes CFTR and SPINK1 mutations

Autoimmune pancreatitis

- Type 1: associated with extrapancreatic manifestations and elevated levels of IgG4-positive cells
- Type 2: low levels of IgG4-positive cells, primarily in the pancreas

Recurrent and severe acute pancreatitis

- Postnecrotic (severe acute pancreatitis)
- Recurrent acute pancreatitis
- Vascular diseases/ischemia
- Postirradiation

Obstructive pancreatitis

- Pancreatic divisum
- Sphincter of Oddi disorders (see Chapter 7)
- Duct obstruction (e.g. by tumor)
- Periampullary duodenal wall cysts
- Post-traumatic pancreatic duct scars

CFTR, cystic fibrosis transmembrane conductance regulator (gene); Ig, immunoglobulin; PRSS1, protease serine 1 (gene); SPINK1, serine protease inhibitor, Kazal type 1 (gene).

Diagnosis

The diagnosis depends on clinical presentation and a combination of functional and radiological investigations, although the latter may appear entirely normal, even in late-stage disease.

Symptoms and signs. About 50% of patients develop pancreatic exocrine and endocrine deficiency some 20 years after disease onset, and about 80% experience pain. Pancreatic exocrine insufficiency occurs when more than 90% of the parenchyma is destroyed; it manifests as steatorrhea and weight loss.

Both chronic pancreatitis and AIP have a variable clinical course, which includes focal masses, strictures of the pancreatic and/or bile duct with subsequent obstruction and dilation (leading to jaundice), and chronic/recurrent pain and weight loss.

Pancreatic exocrine failure. Features include:
- weight loss
- steatorrhea (fatty stool) – more than 7 g fat excreted per day on a normal fat diet
- avoidance of fat
- vitamin deficiency
- peptic ulcer due to loss of bicarbonate secretion (normally produced by the pancreatic ductal cells), and thus loss of buffering capacity against gastric acid arriving in the duodenum from the stomach.

Pancreatic endocrine failure. Features include:
- weight loss
- polydypsia
- polyuria
- diabetic ketoacidosis.

Causes of pain. The pain of chronic pancreatitis is multifactorial in origin, but modern theories principally relate to nerve alterations (Figure 9.2).
- The number and diameter of intra- and interlobular nerve bundles in pancreatic tissue is increased.
- The perineurium is damaged; GAP-43 (growth-associated protein 43, a marker of neural plasticity) is significantly increased in pancreatic nerve fibers.

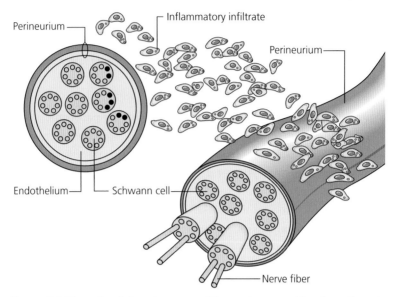

Figure 9.2 The pain of chronic pancreatitis may be caused by disruption of the perineurium and inflammatory infiltrate.

- Levels of neurotransmitters such as calcitonin gene-related peptide and substance P are increased.
- Inflammatory cells interact with the damaged nerves (neuroimmune interactions). Expression of nerve growth factor and tyrosine kinase receptor A is increased and has a significant relationship with pain intensity.
- Pain may be increased as a consequence of local complications such as pseudocysts and biliary tract or duodenal obstruction.
- Pain is also associated with the inability to digest fat properly (malabsorption).
- Older theories include increased intraductal pressure and compartment syndrome.

Laboratory tests

Blood tests. Amylase or lipase levels may be elevated during an acute exacerbation, otherwise they are usually normal. Liver tests may indicate biochemical biliary obstruction. Elevated IgG4 autoantibodies may indicate AIP.

Fecal elastase is a simple test; it is useful if the result is clearly abnormal (< 200 µg/g).

Pancreatolauryl test is a more accurate determinant than fecal elastase, but requires a 3-day complete urine collection.

Secretin test is the best of the functional tests, but is performed only in specialist centers as it requires intubation of the stomach and duodenum and continuous aspiration of pancreatic secretions for 2 hours after stimulation by intravenous secretin.

Imaging

Plain abdominal radiography may show calcifications of the pancreas.

Endoscopic ultrasonography (EUS) is a highly sensitive test for chronic pancreatitis in moderate to severe form (Figure 9.3); a normal EUS correlates well with the absence of chronic pancreatitis. Because of the high sensitivity, minimal or early changes of chronic pancreatitis should be interpreted with caution; overdiagnosis is possible, as there is overlap with age-related changes, and there are more issues with interobserver variability in the case of minimal or equivocal changes.

Contrast-enhanced computed tomography may show ductal abnormalities, pseudocysts or vascular complications. A pancreatic pseudocyst should be differentiated from a pancreatic cystic tumor. CT is very sensitive at detecting calcifications (Figure 9.4).

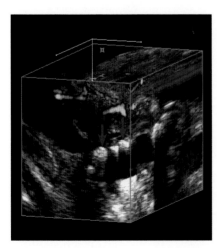

Figure 9.3 Tridimensional (3D) reconstruction of endoscopic ultrasound in a patient with severe chronic pancreatitis showing a dilated common bile duct, as well as a pancreatic duct with multiple calcifications and ductal stones.

95

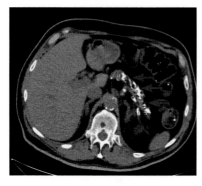

Figure 9.4 Abdominal CT scan showing extensive parenchymal and ductal calcifications in a patient with advanced chronic pancreatitis.

Magnetic resonance cholangiopancreatography may reveal abnormalities in the biliary and pancreatic ducts, such as strictures, dilation and pseudocysts (Figure 9.5).

Tissue diagnosis by endoscopic ultrasonography. EUS-guided fine needle aspiration and EUS-guided core biopsy techniques appear to be attractive options for cytological or tissue diagnosis of chronic pancreatitis. However, the application of these techniques for chronic pancreatitis is still developing (along with concern about complications, especially with EUS-guided core biopsy) and they are not yet used routinely, except for the differentiation of pancreatic adenocarcinoma from pseudotumoral chronic pancreatitis (Figure 9.6).

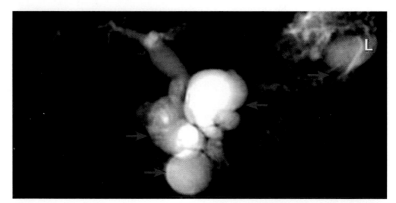

Figure 9.5 Magnetic resonance cholangiopancreatography in advanced chronic pancreatitis showing a double duct sign with obstruction of both the common bile duct and pancreatic duct, as well as multiple pseudocysts at the level of the pancreatic head.

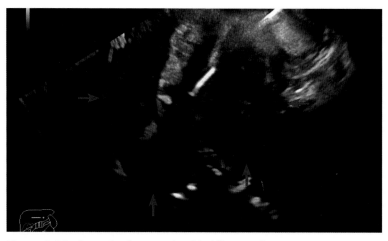

Figure 9.6 Endoscopic ultrasound-guided fine needle aspiration in a patient with pseudotumoral chronic pancreatitis.

Positron emission tomography may not reliably distinguish chronic pancreatitis from pancreatic cancer.

Medical treatment

Elimination of environmental risk factors such as alcohol consumption and tobacco smoking may modify symptoms and, to some extent, the long-term outcome. Before any type of interventional treatment is considered, medical management must be optimized.

The factors governing appropriate fat digestion are complex (Figure 9.7). Fat intake should not be restricted but the patient must take sufficient pancreatic enzyme supplementation with each meal. Replacement of lipase is the key factor; at least 40 to 80 000 lipase units should be divided between meals every day. The addition of a proton pump inhibitor is of particular importance, as this will increase duodenal pH and improve lipase activity. Some pancreatic enzyme products are microencapsulated enteric-coated preparations which prevent acid denaturation of lipase through delayed release.

Other medical treatments include:

- treatment of diabetes
- analgesia
- psychosocial support.

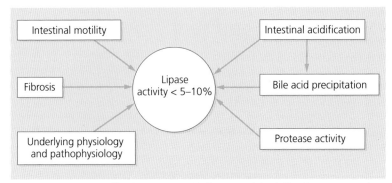

Figure 9.7 Factors affecting pancreatic lipase activity following pancreatic resection.

AIP should be treated with steroids or other immunosuppressive medications.

Patients with intermittent pain appear to have a more favorable disease course. The American Gastroenterological Association has produced guidelines for the management of pain, which can be quite problematic (Figure 9.8). Family and psychosocial support is particularly important. For patients with an alcohol problem it is important that any employment involving alcohol (such as the entertainment industry) is changed.

Endoscopic treatment

Relieving main pancreatic duct obstruction caused by stones and/or strictures requires the use of stents (placed during endoscopic retrograde cholangiopancreatography [ERCP]) and extracorporeal shock wave lithotripsy, but is only applicable to simple strictures and single duct stones. There may be little effect on pain and the techniques do not influence the development of pancreatic insufficiency.

Drainage of the biliary tree. Endoscopic stenting may be used as a temporary measure, but the medium- and long-term success rate is poor. Choice between endoscopic and surgical drainage relies on patient comorbidities and compliance with repeat endoscopic procedures.

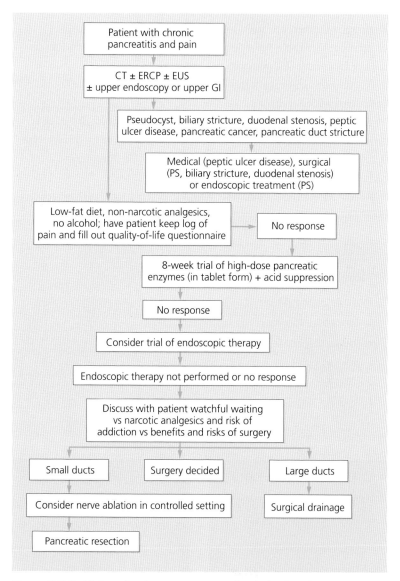

Figure 9.8 Guidelines for the management of pain in chronic pancreatitis developed by the American Gastroenterological Association. CT, computed tomography; ERCP, endoscopic retrograde cholangiopancreatography; EUS, endoscopic ultrasonography; GI, gastrointestinal; PS, pancreatic duct stricture. Adapted from American Gastroenterological Association, 1998.

Drainage of pancreatic pseudocysts. Many pseudocysts resolve spontaneously (Table 9.3); only persisting symptomatic pseudocysts require treatment. Pseudocysts may be drained into the stomach or duodenum using a transmural (usually under EUS guidance; Figure 9.9) or transpapillary technique (during ERCP).

The technical success rate for EUS-guided pseudocyst drainage is around 90–95%, with a morbidity of 15% and mortality of less than 0.25%, which is lower than surgical drainage. The long-term recurrence rate is about 10%.

Relatively simple pseudocysts without parenchymal disease are most suitable for endoscopic treatment.

TABLE 9.3

Factors associated with pseudocyst resolution

- Acute pancreatitis
- Small pseudocysts
- Intrapancreatic pseudocyst
- Pseudocyst of the head of the pancreas
- Persistence < 6 weeks
- Thin pseudocyst wall

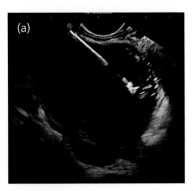
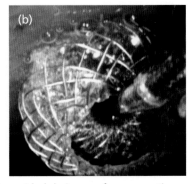

Figure 9.9 Endoscopic ultrasonography-guided drainage of a pancreatic pseudocyst showing (a) initial puncture of the gastric wall and (b) subsequent placement of a double-flanged expandable stent.

Celiac plexus block under EUS guidance or percutaneous routes may be undertaken in some patients, but generally one should not expect long-term pain relief. Limited data comparing the two techniques suggest the EUS-guided route may be more effective. Most clinicians prefer to do a block with steroids and bupivacaine instead of using ablative or sclerosing agents like alcohol. This is because of the higher risk of irreversible complications (e.g neurological), and as any subsequent surgery may be difficult owing to intense fibrosis around major vessels.

Surgical treatment

Bilateral thoracoscopic splanchnicectomy is a minimally invasive thoracic approach that divides the greater, lesser and least splanchnic nerves of the sympathetic system, which carry afferent pain fibers from the pancreas. This procedure provides good short-term pain relief in about 50% of patients – particularly those with no prior intervention – but the benefit is greatly reduced in the long term.

Pancreatic duct drainage procedures. Lateral pancreatojejunostomy requires a dilated duct of at least 6–7 mm diameter and is associated with low mortality (up to 5%) and morbidity. Pain relief is moderate to good in 80% of patients in the short-term, but only 50–60% of patients are pain free at 5 years. There is little effect on pain in patients with advanced chronic pancreatitis.

Drainage of pancreatic pseudocysts. The indications for surgical internal drainage of pancreatic pseudocysts include:
- contraindication or failure of endoscopic and radiological methods
- associated complex pathology, such as an inflammatory mass in the head of the pancreas
- pseudocysts with complex or multiple main pancreatic duct strictures
- pseudocysts with a main bile duct stricture
- left-sided portal hypertension (splenic vein compression/thrombosis) with gastric varices.

The techniques include pseudocystjejunostomy, pseudocystgastrostomy and pseudocystduodenostomy, and have a

101

95–100% success rate, with a long-term recurrence rate of 5%. The operative morbidity is 15%, with a mortality rate of 1–3%, depending on the complexity of the underlying disease.

Bypass of biliary or duodenal obstruction. Biliary stricture occurs in 6% of patients and duodenal obstruction in 1%. Choledochojejunostomy or choledochoduodenostomy are performed for bile duct stricture, and gastrojejunostomy for duodenal obstruction. The success rates are over 98%. Combined obstruction of the pancreatic duct, main bile duct and duodenum requires a resection, or double drainage if this is not possible.

Pancreatic resection achieves the best results for intractable pain in chronic pancreatitis. Long-term pain relief is achieved in 70–95% of patients, but there is a still a mortality of 1–3%. The outcome is better if patients have not been long-term heavy users of opioid analgesia. Various types of surgical procedures have been described.

Pylorus-preserving Whipple partial pancreatoduodenectomy is still valuable if the pancreatic parenchyma is relatively 'soft'; this is the most common procedure and assumes removal of the pancreatic head, gallbladder, duodenum and a portion of the common bile duct, preserving the pylorus and stomach.

Beger operation consists of removal of almost all of the pancreas head, preserving the duodenum, stomach and bile duct. It is appropriate for a dominant inflammatory mass in the head of the pancreas or small duct disease (Figure 9.10).

Frey procedure combines lateral pancreatojejunostomy with the removal of some of the tissue in the head of the pancreas.

Left ('distal') pancreatectomy with spleen preservation is used for dominant left-sided disease.

Total pancreatectomy with preservation of the duodenum and spleen may be indicated for patients with disabling pain for whom previous partial resection has failed or for those with total endocrine and exocrine pancreatic failure.

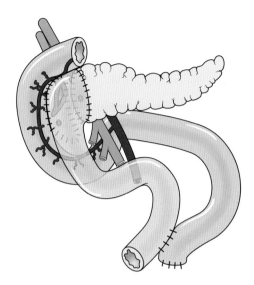

Figure 9.10 Beger operation – duodenum-preserving resection of the head of the pancreas.

Complications

Complications of chronic pancreatitis include:

- abdominal pain (intermittent or continuous – with increased pain during exacerbations); typically the pain is in the epigastrium and the back, and is relieved by flexion
- abdominal mass – mass-forming pancreatitis, pseudotumoral chronic pancreatitis, pseudocysts or pancreatic cancer
- jaundice due to biliary obstruction
- vomiting due to duodenal obstruction
- abdominal distension due to pancreatic ascites
- upper gastrointestinal hemorrhage due to gastric varices
- massive intra-abdominal bleeding due to pseudoaneurysm
- cachexia secondary to pancreatic ductal adenocarcinoma
- diabetes mellitus, in severe cases – sometimes called type III diabetes.

Follow-up

Follow-up consists of frequent (yearly) non-invasive testing by routine laboratory blood tests and transabdominal ultrasound looking for complications such as:

- biliary obstruction and extrahepatic cholestasis
- pancreatic exocrine (total protein, albumin, etc.) and endocrine insufficiency (diabetes)
- steatorrhea.

Many patients lose the support of their friends and family or their employment, especially if the pancreatitis is associated with alcohol consumption.

Patients should lead a healthy lifestyle (low-fat diet, no alcohol and no smoking).

Future trends
- Earlier diagnosis and referral to pancreas treatment centers.
- Genetic counseling and intervention in patients with hereditary and idiopathic chronic pancreatitis.
- Drugs that will modify the progression of the disease.
- Genetically engineered insulin-producing cells.
- Effective secondary screening for pancreatic cancer.
- More effective pain control measures.
- Further refinement of endoscopic and surgical techniques.

Key points – chronic pancreatitis

- The diagnosis must be clearly established by radiological, endoscopic and/or functional tests.
- Risk factors such as smoking and alcohol should be discouraged.
- Medical measures must be optimized.
- Beside medical treatment, severe pain may need endoscopic or surgical intervention.
- Chronic pancreatitis is a risk factor for pancreatic cancer, which may develop within the chronic pancreatitis.

Key references

Aghdassi A, Mayerle J, Kraft M et al. Diagnosis and treatment of pancreatic pseudocysts in chronic pancreatitis. *Pancreas* 2008;36: 105–12.

Andriulli A, Botteri E, Almasio PL et al. Smoking as a cofactor for causation of chronic pancreatitis: a meta-analysis. *Pancreas* 2010;39:1205–10.

Braganza JM, Lee SH, McCloy RF, McMahon MJ. Chronic pancreatitis. *Lancet* 2011;377:1184–97.

Brock C, Nielsen LM, Lelic D, Drewes AM. Pathophysiology of chronic pancreatitis. *World J Gastroenterol* 2013;19:7231–40.

DiMagno MJ, DiMagno EP. Chronic pancreatitis. *Curr Opin Gastroenterol* 2012;28:523–31.

Dumonceau JM, Delhaye M, Tringali A et al. Endoscopic treatment of chronic pancreatitis: European Society of Gastrointestinal Endoscopy (ESGE) Clinical Guideline. *Endoscopy* 2012;44: 784–800.

Dumonceau JM, Macias-Gomez C. Endoscopic management of complications of chronic pancreatitis. *World J Gastroenterol* 2013;19:7308–15.

Finkelberg DL, Sahani D, Deshpande V, Brugge WR. Autoimmune pancreatitis. *N Engl J Med* 2006;355:2670–6.

Gupta V, Toskes P. Diagnosis and management of chronic pancreatitis. *Postgrad Med J* 2005;81:491–7.

Ketwaroo GA, Sheth S. Autoimmune Pancreatitis. *Gastroenterol Rep* 2013;1:27–32.

Klöppel G. Chronic pancreatitis, pseudotumors and other tumor-like lesions. *Mod Pathol* 2007;20(suppl 1):S113–31.

Krasinskas AM, Raina A, Khalid A et al. Autoimmune pancreatitis. *Gastroenterol Clin North Am* 2007;36:239–57.

Perez-Johnston R, Sainani NI, Sahani DV. Imaging of chronic pancreatitis (including groove and autoimmune pancreatitis). *Radiol Clin North Am* 2012;50:447–66.

Poulsen JL, Olesen SS, Malver LP et al. Pain and chronic pancreatitis: a complex interplay of multiple mechanisms. *World J Gastroenterol* 2013;19:7282–91.

Strobel O, Büchler MW, Werner J. Surgical therapy of chronic pancreatitis: indications, techniques and results. *Int J Surg* 2009;7: 305–12.

Yin Z, Sun J, Yin D, Wang J. Surgical treatment strategies in chronic pancreatitis: a meta-analysis. *Arch Surg* 2012;147:961–8.

Genetic predisposition plays a strong part in the clinical manifestation of three types of chronic pancreatitis:

- hereditary pancreatitis
- idiopathic pancreatitis
- alcohol-related pancreatitis.

Hereditary pancreatitis

Hereditary pancreatitis represents a rare cause of chronic pancreatitis and is associated mostly with mutations in the protease serine 1 (*PRSS1*) gene. These mutations often afflict individuals from a very young age (< 10 years), inducing recurrent acute abdominal pain (acute pancreatitis) in over 70%. In addition to *PRSS1* mutations, other mutations, primarily mutations in the serine protease inhibitor Kazal type 1 (*SPINK1*) and cystic fibrosis transmembrane conductance regulator (*CFTR*) genes, are involved in the etiopathogenesis of hereditary pancreatitis.

Patients can have severe episodes of acute recurrent pancreatitis, which lead to chronic pancreatitis with calcifications, and possibly exocrine and endocrine insufficiency. The risk of pancreatic cancer in these patients is higher compared with the general population. By the age of 70 years, 60% of patients with hereditary pancreatitis will develop exocrine insufficiency, including all of the expected symptoms of steatorrhea and weight loss. By this age, 70% will also develop diabetes mellitus, almost all of whom will require insulin. Exocrine and endocrine failure develop in a much higher proportion of patients with hereditary pancreatitis than those with either idiopathic or alcoholic pancreatitis, but the time until failure is longer. About 35% of 70-year-old patients are at risk of pancreatic cancer. This incidence is much higher than with other forms of chronic pancreatitis (around 5%) and compares with an incidence of 1% in the general population.

Idiopathic pancreatitis

Idiopathic pancreatitis occurs in up to 20% of patients with chronic pancreatitis. After exclusion of common etiologic factors (alcohol, occult pancreatic tumor, hypertriglyceridemia, duct obstruction, trauma, pancreas divisum, autoimmune pancreatitis and hyperparathyroidism) as well as hereditary pancreatitis, it has no apparent cause other than a genetic predisposition. There are two types of idiopathic pancreatitis: the most common is early onset (child or young adult), whereas the other occurs in much older patients.

Alcohol-related pancreatitis

About 70% of chronic pancreatitis cases are associated with chronic excess alcohol consumption, but fewer than 10% of known alcoholics develop chronic pancreatitis. Whereas cumulative alcohol consumption is directly related to the development of liver cirrhosis, this is not the case in chronic alcohol-related pancreatitis, which appears to be associated with a lower threshold of total alcohol consumed. About 10% of patients develop both liver cirrhosis and chronic pancreatitis. Inherited genetic factors are clearly involved but are incompletely understood.

Etiology and pathogenesis

The histological and radiological features of these three types of chronic pancreatitis (hereditary, idiopathic and alcohol-related) are indistinguishable.

Inherited abnormal genes play a strong part in the clinical manifestation of the three distinct types of pancreatitis. The genes responsible and their association with the different types of pancreatitis are outlined in Table 10.1. Figure 10.1 shows the mechanisms by which mutation in *PRSS1* and *SPINK1* result in inappropriate trypsin activity within the pancreatic parenchyma. Mutations in *PRSS1* (the trypsinogen gene) result in spontaneous excess self-activation of trypsinogen or resistance to the deactivating enzymes, or both. Once the first line of defense is breached, inactivation of trypsin is not possible if *SPINK1* is mutated.

The CFTR protein moves chloride ions out of the pancreatic ductal

TABLE 10.1

Abnormal genes associated with inherited forms of chronic pancreatitis

Protease serine 1 (*PRSS1*) gene

- Also known as the cationic trypsinogen gene
- Main cause of hereditary pancreatitis
- Autosomal-dominant inheritance
- Located on chromosome 7
- Mutations mainly at codons 122, 29 and 16
- More than 20 mutations have been described
- Mutations of *PRSS1* are found in up to 80% of families with hereditary pancreatitis but are very rare in the general population
- In affected families, the penetrance of the disease is about 80% (the disease is silent in the other 20%)

Cystic fibrosis transmembrane conductance regulator (*CFTR*) gene

- Autosomal-recessive inheritance
- Mutations or polymorphisms found in:
  - up to 5% of the general population
  - up to 20% of patients with alcohol-related chronic pancreatitis
  - over 50% of patients with idiopathic pancreatitis
- Compound heterozygotes are common (different mutations in each of the *CFTR* gene alleles)
- One of more than 2000 different mutations or polymorphisms may be involved

Serine protease inhibitor, Kazal type 1 (*SPINK1*) gene

- Also known as the pancreatic secretory trypsin inhibitor *(PSTI)* gene
- Autosomal-recessive inheritance
- Most common mutation is N34S, found in:
  - 0.5–4% of the general population
  - about 10% of patients with alcohol-related chronic pancreatitis
  - up to 30% of patients with idiopathic pancreatitis
- The N34S mutation may be found clustered in families with a high incidence of pancreatitis, but the disease does not necessarily relate to the presence of the mutation

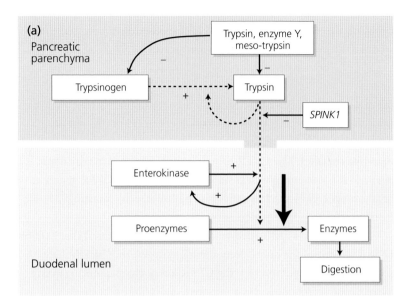

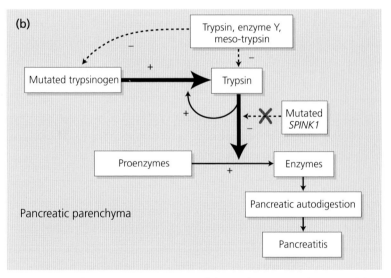

Figure 10.1 Schematic representation of the pathogenesis of pancreatitis secondary to mutations of either the *PRSS1* (trypsinogen) or *SPINK1* genes (Table 10.1). (a) The normal activation mechanism of trypsinogen to trypsin and the regulation of inappropriately activated trypsin. (b) Gene mutations that affect either trypsinogen or *SPINK1* result in inappropriate trypsinogen activation within the pancreatic parenchyma, and thus pancreatitis.

cells into the pancreatic duct lumen in response to secretin hormone stimulation. A large movement of sodium and bicarbonate ions together with a large volume of water molecules accompanies the movement of chloride. This helps to wash the pancreatic enzymes into the duodenal lumen, and the bicarbonate ions counteract the hydrogen ions in the gastric juice entering the duodenum. Thus, the pH of duodenal chyme is raised, which helps to optimize the activity of the digestive enzymes. The CFTR protein is not produced in pancreatic acini, so it is not entirely clear how mutations of the *CFTR* gene also result in pancreatitis that is otherwise pathologically indistinguishable from any other type of pancreatitis.

Pancreatic ducts are loaded with a protein-rich material that cannot be washed out of the ducts. New theories suggest that bicarbonate secretion is regulated through the CFTR anion channel during active bicarbonate secretion, with various gene mutations that might lead to pancreas-specific injury.

Mutations of the chymotrypsin C (caldecrin) gene (*CTRC*) and the calcium-sensing receptor gene (*CASR*) are associated with relatively lower increases in risk for chronic pancreatitis.

Epidemiology

The prevalence of hereditary pancreatitis, at least in northern Europe, has been greatly underestimated; in fact it affects at least one family in every million in the general population.

Diagnosis

The diagnosis, as with all other types of chronic pancreatitis, will depend on clinical presentation and a combination of functional and imaging investigations. The distinction between hereditary pancreatitis and idiopathic chronic pancreatitis requires a careful family history (Figure 10.2). For a diagnosis of hereditary pancreatitis, there should be at least two first-degree relatives in two or more generations with proven chronic pancreatitis. Genetic testing of symptomatic children of an individual with the condition may be considered as this may help clinical diagnosis and management. The detection of a *PRSS1* mutation will clinch the diagnosis, but it must be remembered that

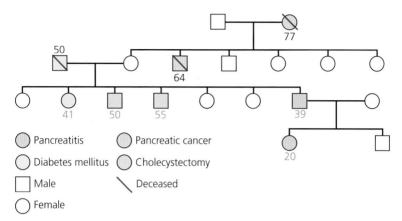

Figure 10.2 A typical family tree of a patient with hereditary pancreatitis.

about 20% of patients do not have a mutation of this gene.

The nature of the abdominal pain seen in hereditary pancreatitis is commonly misdiagnosed in children and young adults; this fact, coupled with the reduced penetrance, often leads to clinical confusion and a failure to identify the existence of close relatives with pancreatitis.

It is vital that patients undergo appropriate genetic counseling before any genetic tests are undertaken. A positive genetic test may help in the future management of any symptomatic children. Patients with idiopathic chronic pancreatitis are at high risk of having a *CFTR* mutation; this may have significant implications for people planning to have children, particularly in areas where there are many carriers of the mutated *CFTR* gene in the general population. This is because there will be an increased risk of parenting a child with cystic fibrosis (an autosomal-recessive condition) caused by the inheritance of two mutated *CFTR* genes, one from each parent.

Symptoms and signs. The typical presentation is an acute attack of epigastric pain, which often results in hospitalization. Recurrent acute attacks of pain eventually merge into chronic pancreatitis, with continuous pain and ultimately a steady loss of pancreatic function.

The median age for presentation for hereditary pancreatitis is around 12 years, but presentation is earlier in children with an *R122H*   111 mutation (10 years) than in other patients (15 years). Most patients present by the age of 20 years and 95% by the age of 50 years. In the absence of a family history, the diagnosis of hereditary pancreatitis is commonly missed. Typically, children are thought to have a viral infection, Crohn's disease or psychosomatic pain (periodic syndrome). Young adults with hereditary or idiopathic chronic pancreatitis may be diagnosed with celiac disease or irritable bowel syndrome. The median age for presentation for early-onset idiopathic chronic pancreatitis is 20–30 years, 35–45 years for alcohol-related chronic pancreatitis and 60 years for late-onset idiopathic chronic pancreatitis.

Treatment

The treatment of hereditary pancreatitis is at first identical to that of other forms of chronic pancreatitis. Alcohol consumption and tobacco smoking are both independent risk factors for chronic pancreatitis and pancreatic cancer, and should therefore be strongly discouraged.

As with other forms of chronic pancreatitis, about 30% of patients will require active intervention by endoscopy and/or surgery because of local pancreatic complications or intractable pain. From the age of 40 years, patients with hereditary pancreatitis should be counseled regarding regular secondary screening for the detection of pancreatic cancer. Screening is an evolving field and international guidelines state that it should only take place at major regional pancreas centers using both MRI and endoscopic ultrasonography.

In appropriate cases, prophylactic total pancreatectomy may be offered, especially if there is complete endocrine and exocrine failure in conjunction with chronic abdominal pain that is difficult to control.

Future trends

- Routine genetic counseling and gene testing in regional pancreas centers for all families with hereditary and idiopathic pancreatitis.
- Discovery of additional genes to explain nearly all cases of hereditary pancreatitis.
- New treatments to modify progression of the disease.
- Improved methods of secondary screening to reduce deaths from pancreatic cancer.

Key points – hereditary pancreatitis

- Hereditary pancreatitis is an autosomal disease mainly caused by protease serine 1 (*PRSS1*) mutations with 80% penetrance.
- Patients with idiopathic chronic pancreatitis are likely to carry cystic fibrosis transmembrane conductance regulator (*CFTR*) mutations in one or both alleles of the gene (compound heterozygotes).
- Children and young adults are often misdiagnosed with other gastrointestinal diseases.
- There is a lifetime risk of pancreatic cancer (35%), as well as a high risk of diabetes mellitus and exocrine insufficiency.
- Patients should undergo genetic counseling prior to genetic testing, and from the age of 40 years patients should be offered secondary screening for cancer in a regional pancreas cancer center.
- Alcohol and tobacco consumption should be strongly discouraged.

Key references

Ballard DD, Flueckiger JR, Fogel EL et al. Evaluating adults with idiopathic pancreatitis for genetic predisposition: higher prevalence of abnormal results with use of complete gene sequencing. *Pancreas* 2015;44:116–21.

Braganza JM, Dormandy TL. Micronutrient therapy for chronic pancreatitis: rationale and impact. *JOP* 2010;11:99–112.

Canto MI, Harinck F, Hruban RH et al. International Cancer of the Pancreas Screening (CAPS) Consortium summit on the management of patients with increased risk for familial pancreatic cancer. *Gut* 2013;62:339–47.

Ceppa EP, Pitt HA, Hunter JL et al. Hereditary pancreatitis: endoscopic and surgical management. *J Gastrointest Surg* 2013;17:847–56.

Cohn JA, Friedman KJ, Noone PG et al. Relation between mutations of the cystic fibrosis gene and idiopathic pancreatitis. *N Engl J Med* 1998;339:653–8.

Langer P, Kann PH, Fendrich V. Five years of prospective screening of high-risk individuals from families with familial pancreatic cancer. *Gut* 2009;58:1410–18.

McFaul CD, Greenhalf W, Earl J et al. Anticipation in familial pancreatic cancer. *Gut* 2006;55: 252–8.

Noone PG, Zhou Z, Silverman LM et al. Cystic fibrosis gene mutations and pancreatitis risk: relation to epithelial ion transport and trypsin inhibitor gene mutations. *Gastroenterology* 2001;121:1310–19.

Patel MR, Eppolito AL, Willingham FF. Hereditary pancreatitis for the endoscopist. *Therap Adv Gastroenterol* 2013;6:169–79.

Pelaez-Luna M, Robles-Diaz G, Canizales-Quinteros S, Tusié-Luna MT. PRSS1 and SPINK1 mutations in idiopathic chronic and recurrent acute pancreatitis. *World J Gastroenterol* 2014;20:11788–92.

Pfützer RH, Barmada MM, Brunskill AP et al. SPINK1/PSTI polymorphisms act as disease modifiers in familial and idiopathic chronic pancreatitis. *Gastroenterology* 2000;119:615–23.

Poruk KE, Firpo MA, Adler DG, Mulvihill SJ. Screening for pancreatic cancer: why, how, and who? *Ann Surg* 2013;257:17–26.

Rebours V, Boutron-Ruault MC, Schnee M et al. The natural history of hereditary pancreatitis: a national series. *Gut* 2009;58:97–103.

Rebours V, Lévy P, Ruszniewski P. An overview of hereditary pancreatitis. *Dig Liver Dis* 2012;44:8–15.

Whitcomb DC. Genetic risk factors for pancreatic disorders. *Gastroenterology* 2013;144:1292–302.

Witt H, Luck W, Hennies HC et al. Mutations in the gene encoding the serine protease inhibitor, Kazal type 1 are associated with chronic pancreatitis. *Nature Genet* 2000;25:213–16.

Etiology and pathogenesis

The term pancreatic cancer usually refers to common pancreatic ductal adenocarcinoma, although there is a large variety of other exocrine solid tumor types (Table 11.1) with varying prognoses.

Pancreatic cancer usually arises in the head of the pancreas (80%) and less commonly in the body (15%) or tail (5%). Other tumors that arise in the pancreas, or in close proximity to it, are part of the differential diagnosis in a patient with suspected pancreatic adenocarcinoma:

- pancreatic neuroendocrine tumors
- pancreatic lymphoma
- metastatic tumors
- adenocarcinoma of the ampulla of Vater
- intrapancreatic bile duct adenocarcinoma
- duodenal adenocarcinoma.

Pancreatic adenocarcinoma usually has its origin in precursor lesions termed pancreatic intraepithelial neoplasia, which are graded

TABLE 11.1

Common solid exocrine epithelial tumors of the pancreas

Benign tumors

- Hamartoma

Borderline tumors

- Solid pseudopapillary tumor

Malignant tumors

- Ductal adenocarcinoma
- Signet ring cell carcinoma
- Adenosquamous carcinoma
- Anaplastic carcinoma
- Mixed ductal endocrine carcinoma
- Osteoclast-like giant cell tumor
- Acinar cell carcinoma
- Pancreatoblastoma

from 1 to 3. Once the lesions progress to invasive carcinoma there is a strong desmoplastic reaction that impedes both diagnosis and treatment as a result of the decreased penetration of chemotherapeutic agents inside tumors.

The *KRAS* oncogene is frequently altered in pancreatic adenocarcinomas. It can be activated by various factors and is involved in pancreatic cell transformation, tumor formation and progression. Other somatic mutations have been reported, including alterations of several tumor suppressor genes, such as *CDKN2A* (p16; cell cycle regulation), *TP53* (p53; cellular stress response) and *DPC4* (SMAD4), which modifies cellular signaling of the tumor growth factor-β pathway.

Epidemiology and risk factors

Pancreatic adenocarcinoma is one of the most common causes of death from cancer in westernized countries. Worldwide there are approximately 250 000 new cases each year: 70 000 in Europe and 32 000 in the USA. The overall crude incidence of pancreatic adenocarcinoma is approximately 10 per 100 000 people; the peak incidence is in the 65–75-year age group. Tobacco smoking is the major risk factor. The second most important risk factor is a familial background (5–10%).

Familial pancreatic cancer is rare, although germline mutations of the *BRCA2* gene are found in 10–20% of such families. Other families have a combination of pancreatic cancer and melanoma in which there are germline mutations of the gene $p16^{Ink4a}$. Furthermore, a variety of familial pancreatic syndromes have a significantly increased risk of pancreatic cancer:
- Peutz–Jeghers syndrome
- familial breast and ovarian cancer
- familial atypical multiple mole melanoma
- hereditary non-polyposis colon cancer
- ataxia telangiectasia
- Li–Fraumeni syndrome
- familial adenomatous polyposis
- cystic fibrosis.

The risk of pancreatic adenocarcinoma is increased about fivefold in chronic pancreatitis and 40-fold in hereditary pancreatitis. There is also an association with diabetes mellitus, especially in older patients.

Diagnosis

Symptoms and signs of pancreatic cancer are shown in Table 11.2. In the case of tumors of the head of the pancreas, painless obstructive jaundice (jaundice with dark urine and pale stools) commonly occurs but the presentation is usually insidious. Weight loss, nausea, vomiting, and abdominal and back pain can also be suggestive of pancreatic head cancer, although they are more frequently encountered in body and tail tumors. As a result of the location, symptoms appear earlier in the head of the pancreas, while the evolution is often insidious until late stages in body and tail lesions.

Pancreatic cancer should be suspected in any patient (over 40 years of age) with unresolving epigastric symptoms.

Functioning pancreatic neuroendocrine tumors have their own particular modes of presentation (see Chapter 12).

Laboratory tests

Blood tests should be carried out for anemia, clotting profile, proteins and liver function.

Serum cancer antigen (CA) 19.9 is a useful tumor marker, but not all pancreatic adenocarcinomas have elevated CA 19.9. It can be elevated in benign disease and in the presence of obstructive jaundice or chronic pancreatitis.

Imaging

Radiology. Cancers in the head of the pancreas will cause dilation of both the main bile duct and the main pancreatic duct (97%), giving rise to the classic 'double-duct' radiological sign (visualized by transabdominal ultrasound, CT or MRI). Pancreatic adenocarcinomas are relatively hypovascular, whereas neuroendocrine tumors are hypervascular.

Transabdominal ultrasonography should be undertaken as an initial first step.

TABLE 11.2

Symptoms and signs of pancreatic adenocarcinoma

Symptoms	Signs
• painless jaundice and pale-colored stools	• jaundice
• pruritus secondary to jaundice	• scratch marks secondary to jaundice
• fatigue	• multiple bruises (ecchymoses) secondary to impaired clotting
• weight loss	
• back pain (constant, nagging, worse lying down, eased by bending forward and sleeping in sitting position)	• hepatomegaly
	• palpable gallbladder (Courvoisier's sign)
• vague dyspepsia or abdominal discomfort	• cachexia
• anorexia	• left supraclavicular (Virchow's) node enlargement (Troisier's sign)
• constipation (reduced food intake)	• anemia
• steatorrhea (fatty stools)	• abdominal mass
• late-onset diabetes mellitus without risk factors for diabetes	• metastasis at the umbilicus (Sister Joseph's sign)
	• ascites
• acute pancreatitis of unknown cause	• venous gangrene of the lower limbs
• chronic pancreatitis	• migratory thrombophlebitis
• acute cholangitis	
• vomiting (due to duodenal obstruction)	
• deep vein thrombosis	

Transabdominal ultrasound can be used to identify a dilated extrahepatic main bile duct as well as perhaps the primary pancreatic tumor (Figure 11.1) and large liver metastases, if present. This should never be used alone to exclude a pancreatic cancer. In developed countries, transabdominal ultrasound is being used less and less when a

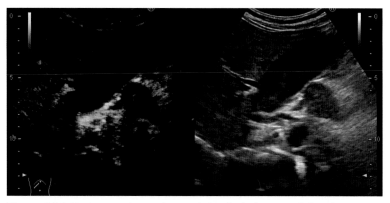

Figure 11.1 Contrast-enhanced transabdominal ultrasound showing a hypovascular pancreatic tumor, highly suggestive of adenocarcinoma.

pancreatic cancer is strongly suspected, and physicians directly order a CT scan of the abdomen as the next step. There are certainly geographic variations in the use of transabdominal ultrasound as the initial test for imaging the pancreas when a pancreatic cancer is suspected.

Contrast-enhanced computed tomography is the examination of choice for diagnosis and staging for resectability, provided that dedicated pancreatic protocols and latest state-of-the-art multidetector scanners are used (Figure 11.2). Enlargement of lymph nodes per se is a poor prognostic indicator. Portal or splenic venous involvement has become less relevant for surgical resection, while arterial encasement or involvement of the celiac artery and/or superior mesenteric artery is a very important factor in determining resectability. Although

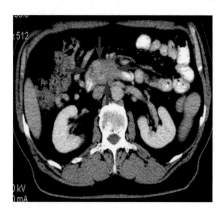

Figure 11.2 Contrast-enhanced CT scan in a patient with pancreatic adenocarcinoma.

dynamic contrast-enhanced CT has less accuracy than endoscopic ultrasonography (EUS) for detecting small tumors (less than 2 cm), for staging purposes CT is still recommended. CT may be supplemented by EUS, MRI and laparoscopy.

Magnetic resonance imaging has similar diagnostic and staging accuracies to CT and is frequently used in conjunction with magnetic resonance cholangiopancreatography.

Magnetic resonance cholangiopancreatography may enhance diagnosis by revealing a double duct sign (dilation of both the common bile duct and pancreatic duct; Figure 11.3).

Endoscopic ultrasonography is highly sensitive for the detection of small tumors (Figure 11.4), and even small lesions (< 10 mm) can be biopsied under EUS guidance. EUS is also useful in staging and is

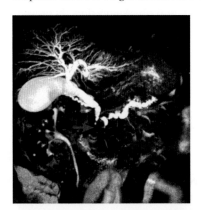

Figure 11.3 Magnetic resonance cholangiopancreatography with 3D reconstructions showing a double duct sign with dilation of the common bile duct, gallbladder and intrahepatic bile ducts, as well as the pancreatic duct.

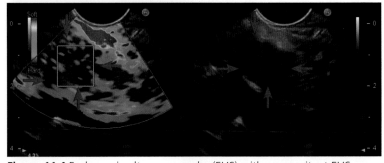

Figure 11.4 Endoscopic ultrasonography (EUS) with concomitant EUS elastography depicting a small pancreatic head adenocarcinoma in close contact with the splenomesenteric confluence.

helpful as the next step in evaluating a potentially resectable or borderline resectable lesion on CT scan. When a CT scan does not show a tumor or is borderline for the presence of a small pancreatic adenocarcinoma (< 1–2 cm), many studies have shown that EUS should be the next test to confirm or exclude the presence of a small pancreatic tumor.

Endoscopic retrograde cholangiopancreatography (ERCP) is important for the diagnosis of ampullary and duodenal tumors as there is direct visualization of the major papilla, allowing the possibility of direct biopsy; brush cytology of the bile and pancreatic ducts may also be undertaken. Nevertheless, ERCP should no longer be used as a pure diagnostic technique (because of the risk of pancreatitis), and is mostly used for the preoperative drainage of the common bile duct in jaundiced patients.

Laparoscopy, including laparoscopic ultrasonography, can detect occult metastatic lesions in the liver and peritoneal cavity and is an important adjunct to CT and EUS for staging at many centers.

Positron-emission tomography (PET) is not routinely used in the diagnosis and staging of pancreatic cancer. However, PET in combination with CT or MRI may play an important role in the future for the staging of pancreatic cancer and patient stratification.

Tissue diagnosis may be obtained by brushings during ERCP or fine needle aspirations (FNA) obtained percutaneously or by EUS. However, EUS-guided FNA is the preferred method for tissue diagnosis and has a higher accuracy than ERCP with brush cytology. Preoperative tissue diagnosis may not always be needed in a resectable pancreatic mass if the symptoms, signs, laboratory data and imaging are classic for pancreatic cancer in an otherwise surgically fit patient. However, when a preoperative tissue diagnosis is required in a potentially resectable pancreatic mass, EUS-guided FNA should be the preferred route on account of the lower potential risk of peritoneal seeding, the shorter needle tract and the inclusion of the needle track in the resection specimen (in pancreatic head tumors). Tissue diagnosis may be needed in borderline resectable pancreatic tumors if the patient is to undergo preoperative neoadjuvant chemotherapy or chemoradiation therapy before surgery.

Differential diagnosis. In the case of solid lesions, the principal differential diagnoses are mass-forming (pseudotumoral) chronic pancreatitis and periampullary tumors (tumors of the intrapancreatic bile duct, ampulla of Vater and duodenum, and 'indeterminate' tumors).

Secondary screening

None of the above diagnostic tests is routinely recommended for screening of the general population, as the overall incidence of pancreatic cancer is low and these tests are considered too expensive for mass screening. Emerging data show that EUS and MRI may be used for secondary screening of high-risk groups, such as those at risk of familial pancreatic cancer. Recent studies have suggested that EUS and MRI are the preferred tests for screening high-risk groups as they detect more lesions than CT and with no radiation involved.

Palliative treatment

The majority of patients present with advanced disease and have an overall median survival of less than 6 months, and a 5-year survival rate of up to 5%. Up to 10–20% of patients undergo pancreatic resection, with an overall median survival of 11–20 months, and a 5-year survival rate of 7–25%; virtually all patients die within 7 years of surgery.

According to published guidelines, all patients with pancreatic cancer must be treated in a specialist high-volume center by a multidisciplinary team (Figure 11.5). Once the diagnosis is made or strongly suspected, the next objective is to stage the disease. If the tumor is resectable and there are no metastases then resection should be undertaken. If resection is not possible then non-surgical treatment should be undertaken.

Stenting of the obstructed biliary tree. ERCP is the preferred method for drainage and stenting of an obstructed biliary tree to relieve jaundice. The stent is retrogradely inserted through the biliary stricture; expandable metallic stents are preferable. If ERCP fails, or is not considered feasible because of the anatomy of the obstruction (or obstruction from the tumor), percutaneous transhepatic

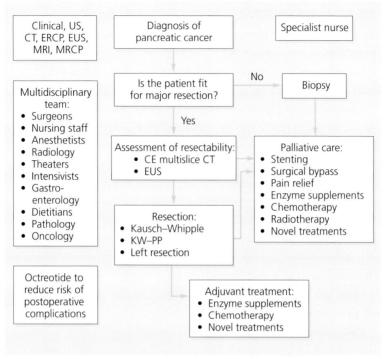

Figure 11.5 Algorithm for the management of patients with pancreatic cancer. CE, contrast-enhanced; CT, computed tomography; ERCP, endoscopic retrograde cholangiopancreatography; EUS, endoscopic ultrasonography; KW-PP, Kausch–Whipple partial pancreatoduodenectomy; MRCP, magnetic resonance cholangiopancreatography; US, ultrasonography. Adapted from Ghaneh et al. Pancreatic cancer. In: Williams C, ed. *Evidence-based Oncology.* London: BMJ Books, 2002; 247–72.

cholangiography is a viable option (antegrade insertion into the stricture). EUS-guided biliary drainage has also become a viable option for failed biliary drainage via ERCP.

Surgical bypass. In younger, fitter patients, biliary bypass may be preferred as blockage of stents is avoided. If duodenal obstruction is determined by tumor invasion, the duodenum may also be bypassed with a gastrojejunostomy.

Pain relief is not easy. A pain team may be needed to advise on the use of opiates, celiac plexus block by an EUS-guided route or bilateral transthoracic sympathectomy.

Enzyme supplements are essential, as the main pancreatic duct is usually blocked, leading to pancreatic exocrine insufficiency.

Chemotherapy. Current treatment options for patients with locally advanced or metastatic cancer include either FOLFIRINOX (a combination regimen consisting of folinic acid [leucovorin], fluorouracil [5-FU], irinotecan and oxaliplatin), gemcitabine, or gemcitabine and albumin-bound nab-paclitaxel. Further options include gemcitabine and erlotinib (an epidermal growth factor inhibitor) or capecitabine.

For second-line therapy, a fluoropyrimidine-based regimen is used for patients previously treated with a gemcitabine-based regimen, or a gemcitabine-based regimen is used for patients previously treated with a fluoropyrimidine-based regimen.

Many trials are under way to find chemotherapy treatments that will improve survival.

Radiotherapy in conjunction with chemotherapy may be helpful in controlling pain in patients with locally advanced disease. However, it is not clear if survival is better than with chemotherapy alone. Some centers have pioneered and established the approach of preoperative chemoradiation followed by surgery in borderline resectable patients to improve survival. This approach is not universally adopted at this time.

Curative surgical treatment

The overall mortality for major pancreatic resections is less than 5% in large centers but is much higher otherwise. Postoperative morbidity is high (30–40%), and patients require high-dependency care for at least the first 24 hours after surgery. Preoperative biliary drainage may be used before surgery to relieve jaundice in cases with cholangitis and fever.

There is increasing evidence of the benefit of neoadjuvant therapy in borderline resectable patients. Current regimens include chemotherapy with FOLFIRINOX, or gemcitabine and albumin-bound paclitaxel, as well as chemoradiotherapy in selected reference centers.

A number of different types of surgery have been described.

Whipple partial pancreatoduodenectomy was once the standard procedure for tumors in the head of the pancreas and is still appropriate for large tumors and those close to the pylorus.

Pylorus-preserving partial pancreatoduodenectomy is largely replacing the Whipple procedure as it does not involve removal of the gastric antrum and pylorus.

Left (distal) partial pancreatectomy includes a splenectomy and is reserved for tumors in the tail of the pancreas.

Total pancreatectomy is reserved for large tumors.

Enucleation is a local resection and is used for small benign neuroendocrine tumors (without metastases) – essentially insulinoma.

Complications following major pancreatic surgery occur in around 30% of patients and require close monitoring (Table 11.3).

TABLE 11.3

Complications of major pancreatic surgery

Respiratory complications	10%
Cardiovascular complications	10%
Pancreatic fistula	10%
Delayed gastric emptying	10%
Bleeding	5%
Wound infection	5%
Intra-abdominal abscess	5%
Mortality	1–5%
Reoperation rate	5–10%
Reoperative mortality	10–30%

Adjuvant treatment

Adjuvant treatment following pancreatic resection is frequently used and consists of chemotherapy with or without the use of radiation. Treatment should be started within 12 weeks after surgery and should include either fluoropyrimidine- or gemcitabine-based chemoradiation, or chemotherapy alone, followed by maintenance 5-FU or gemcitabine. Metastatic sites may also be palliated with radiotherapy.

Future trends

- Improved methods for early diagnosis to improve survival in this very lethal cancer.
- Improved chemotherapy regimens to improve survival in locally advanced and metastatic patients.
- Centralization of treatment in reference centers with multidisciplinary teams.
- Better definition of high-risk patients for inclusion in screening programs using MRI and EUS.
- Use of PET in conjunction with CT/MRI (fusion PET-CT/MRI). This is an evolving technique that measures the metabolism in tumor cells.
- Individual treatment based on the molecular characteristics of each tumor and the pharmacogenomic constitution of the patient.
- Novel biological therapies and cancer vaccination.
- Anticachexia drugs.
- Improved methods of pain control.

Key points – pancreatic adenocarcinoma

- Pancreatic cancer should be suspected in any patient (over 40 years of age) with unresolving epigastric symptoms.
- Patients with pancreatic adenocarcinoma must be managed by a multidisciplinary team in a high-volume regional pancreas cancer center.
- Accurate detection and staging are based on CT and may be supplemented by endoscopic ultrasonography (EUS), MRI and laparoscopy.
- If the cancer is not resectable, symptoms may be relieved with EUS-guided celiac plexus neurolysis and non-surgical treatment consisting of chemotherapy (e.g. gemcitabine or fluoropyrimidine combinations) and pain management.
- In borderline resectable patients, preoperative neoadjuvant chemotherapy and radiation can be considered.
- Adjuvant chemotherapy is used systematically following resection.

Key references

Bhutani MS. Endoscopic ultrasonography – new developments and interesting trends. *Endoscopy* 2004;36:950–6.

Canto MI, Harinck F, Hruban RH et al. International Cancer of the Pancreas Screening (CAPS) Consortium summit on the management of patients with increased risk for familial pancreatic cancer. *Gut* 2013;62:339–47.

di Magliano MP, Logsdon CD. Roles for KRAS in pancreatic tumor development and progression. *Gastroenterology* 2013;144:1220–9.

Harinck F, Konings IC, Kluijt I et al. A multicentre comparative prospective blinded analysis of EUS and MRI for screening of pancreatic cancer in high-risk individuals. *Gut* 2016;65:1505–13.

Hines OJ, Reber HA. Pancreatic surgery. *Curr Opin Gastroenterol* 2009;25:460–5.

Kim EJ, Simeone DM. Advances in pancreatic cancer. *Curr Opin Gastroenterol* 2011;27:460–6.

Krejs GJ. Pancreatic cancer: epidemiology and risk factors. *Dig Dis* 2010;28:355–8.

Rijkers AP, Valkema R, Duivenvoorden HJ, van Eijck CH. Usefulness of F-18-fluorodeoxyglucose positron emission tomography to confirm suspected pancreatic cancer: a meta-analysis. *Eur J Surg Oncol* 2014;40:794-804.

Ryan DP, Hong TS, Bardeesy N. Pancreatic adenocarcinoma. *N Engl J Med* 2014;371:1039–49.

Săftoiu A, Vilmann P. Role of endoscopic ultrasound in the diagnosis and staging of pancreatic cancer. *J Clin Ultrasound* 2009;37:1–17.

Shrikhande SV, Barreto SG, Goel M, Arya S. Multimodality imaging of pancreatic ductal adenocarcinoma: a review of the literature. *HPB (Oxford)* 2012;14:658–68.

Tempero MA, Malafa MP, Behrman SW et al. Pancreatic adenocarcinoma, version 2.2014. *J Natl Compr Canc Netw* 2014;12:1083–93.

Walker EJ, Ko AH. Beyond first-line chemotherapy for advanced pancreatic cancer: an expanding array of therapeutic options? *World J Gastroenterol* 2014;20:2224–36.

Wood LD, Hruban RH. Pathology and molecular genetics of pancreatic neoplasms. *Cancer J* 2012;18:492–501.

Yusuf TE, Bhutani MS. Differentiating pancreatic cancer from pseudotumorous chronic pancreatitis. *Curr Gastroenterol Rep* 2002;4:135–9.

Unusual tumors of the pancreas and ampulla of Vater

A variety of tumors arise in close proximity to or within the pancreas that require special consideration and need to be differentiated from pancreatic ductal adenocarcinoma (Table 12.1).

Ampullary, bile duct and duodenal tumors

Etiology and pathogenesis. Cancers of the ampulla of Vater, the intrapancreatic bile duct and duodenum are all adenocarcinomas and often present in a manner similar to pancreatic cancer. Bile duct cancers are also called cholangiocarcinomas, although this term is

TABLE 12.1

Unusual tumors of or around the pancreas

Solid tumors arising close to the pancreas

- Adenocarcinoma of the ampulla of Vater
- Intrapancreatic bile duct adenocarcinoma
- Duodenal adenocarcinoma

Unusual tumors of the pancreas

Solid tumors	Cystic tumors
Pancreatic neuroendocrine tumors	Serous cystadenoma
Pancreatic lymphoma (as an isolated site)	Mucinous cystadenoma
Metastasis to the pancreas (as an isolated site)	Mucinous cystadenocarcinoma
Other rare tumors of the pancreas	Intraductal papillary mucinous neoplasms

usually reserved for more proximal bile duct tumors. All of these tumors progress from a small benign adenoma through to invasive adenocarcinoma, although most are only detected at the cancerous stage. Ampullary tumors arise from the common channel of the ampulla of Vater as benign adenomas and progress as tubulovillous adenomas before becoming adenocarcinomas. Two pathological types of ampullary cancer have been described (intestinal versus pancreaticobiliary), with important consequences for patients' prognosis. Duodenal tumors also commence as adenomas before progressing to invasive adenocarcinoma. The long-term survival of patients with these cancers is better than that for pancreatic ductal adenocarcinoma (Figure 12.1).

Epidemiology and risk factors. Ampullary tumors are relatively common (around 1 per 100 000 in the general population), whereas bile duct cancer is much less common and duodenal cancer is rare.

The incidence of duodenal tumors is increased in patients with familial adenomatous polyposis and also Peutz–Jeghers syndrome.

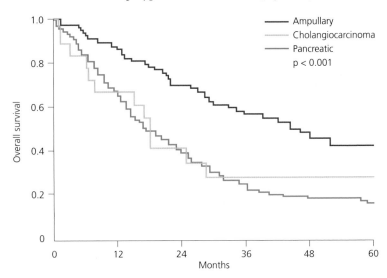

Figure 12.1 Tumor-specific overall survival curves for a cohort of 346 patients treated for periampullary adenocarcinoma by pancreaticoduodenectomy. From Hatzaras et al., 2010, with permission.

Diagnosis

Symptoms and signs. These tumors often present in a manner similar to pancreatic cancer, with obstructive jaundice and weight loss. Patients with an ampullary tumor may also present with intermittent jaundice or acute pancreatitis. Patients with duodenal cancer present with iron-deficiency anemia secondary to occult upper gastrointestinal blood loss.

Clinical presentation. All three tumor types may mimic pancreatic cancer and vice versa.

- Pancreatic cancer may invade into or ulcerate the ampulla, giving the appearance of an ampullary cancer. Ampullary cancer will invade the duodenum and pancreatic parenchyma, mimicking pancreatic cancer.
- Pancreatic cancer may invade and ulcerate the duodenum, giving the appearance of a duodenal cancer. Invasion of the pancreas is typical of a duodenal cancer.
- Bile duct cancer may invade the main pancreatic duct, giving rise to the classic double-duct sign of pancreatic cancer; the converse applies to 95% of pancreatic cancers arising in the head or uncinate process of the pancreas.

Imaging and biopsy. Ampullary and duodenal tumors may be visualized by endoscopic retrograde cholangiopancreatography (ERCP) or endoscopic ultrasonography (EUS). Brush cytology of the bile duct may also be undertaken for bile duct strictures using ERCP. Invasive adenocarcinomas usually arise deep within an ampullary tumor. For this reason, endoscopic sphincterotomy through the ampullary tumor needs to be performed and biopsies taken from deep within the tumor.

Treatment. Ampullary adenomas can be treated by local ampullectomy using a transduodenal approach or by endoscopic excision. Endoscopic snare papillectomy should be accompanied by pancreatic and bile duct stent placement in order to reduce procedure-related complications. A pancreas-preserving total duodenectomy can be used to treat dysplastic duodenal polyps or benign adenomas, especially in patients with familial adenomatous polyposis.

For cancers of the ampulla, bile duct or duodenum, the treatment of choice is a Whipple pancreatoduodenectomy. The 5-year survival rates for completely resected tumors are about 50%, 30% and 25% for cancers of the ampulla, bile duct and duodenum, respectively. Unlike pancreatic cancer, long-term cure is possible in a large proportion of patients with these cancers (see Figure 12.1).

Ampullary tumors tend to be slow growing, so endoscopic stenting can provide good medium-to-long-term palliation in advanced patients. The role of chemoradiation or chemotherapy for these cancers in either the adjuvant or advanced setting is not established.

Pancreatic neuroendocrine tumors

Etiology and pathogenesis. Pancreatic neuroendocrine tumors (pNETs) arise from cells in the islet of Langerhans or enterochromaffin-like cells. In contrast to most other tumors of the pancreas, these tumors tend to be highly vascular, a feature that is important in making a radiological diagnosis.

The tumors may be functioning (Table 12.2), with the ability to secrete peptides and neuroamines (some of which cause specific clinical syndromes), or they may be non-functioning. They may be sporadic in nature (non-inherited) or be part of an inherited neuroendocrine neoplasia syndrome.

Epidemiology and risk factors. The prevalence is around 2–4 per 100 000 in the general population. Nevertheless, this is a heterogeneous group of tumors and the incidence varies according to each specific pNET. Non-functional pNETs are the most frequent entity, being twice as frequent as insulinomas. Insulinomas have an incidence of 1–4 per 1 million people. These are followed by gastrinomas, glucagonomas, vasoactive intestinal polypeptide tumors (VIPomas), somatostatinomas, etc.

Several autosomal dominant diseases are associated with pNETs, including multiple endocrine neoplasia (MEN) type-1, von Hippel-Lindau (VHL) syndrome, von Recklinghausen disease (neurofibromatosis 1) and, rarely, tuberous sclerosis. MEN type-1 is seen in less than 5% of patients with pNETs.

TABLE 12.2

Functioning pancreatic neuroendocrine tumors

- Insulinoma
- Gastrinoma (frequently found in the duodenum)
- Vasoactive intestinal polypeptide tumor (VIPoma) (secretes VIP)
- Somatostatinoma
- Glucagonoma
- Growth hormone-releasing hormone (GHRH)oma (secretes GHRH)
- Adrenocorticotropic hormone (ACTH)oma (secretes ACTH)
- Carcinoid tumor (occurs in the ampulla of Vater)
- Pancreatic polypeptide tumor (PPoma)
- Other rare functioning tumors (secrete luteinizing hormone, rennin, insulin-like growth factor, erythropoietin etc.)

Source: North American Neuroendocrine Tumor Society (NANETS) consensus guidelines.

Symptoms and signs. Both functioning and non-functioning pNETs secrete various substances that do not determine specific hormonal syndromes, such as chromogranin, neuron-specific enolase, neurotensin, ghrelin and subunits of human chorionic gonadotropin. Patients with a suspected pNET require a full hormone screen, which should include chromogranin A and B levels, which are frequently elevated in non-functioning NETs. Specific hormone immunohistochemistry of a resected specimen will confirm the type of functioning NET and distinguish this from a non-functioning NET.

Insulinoma. The classic presentation is Whipple's triad:
- signs and symptoms of hypoglycemia with neuroglycopenic changes (confusion, altered consciousness)
- low blood glucose level at the time signs and symptoms occur
- disappearance of the signs and symptoms when blood glucose levels are raised.

Typically, faintness, fatigue or even coma occurs with fasting (or vigorous exercise) and is relieved rapidly by eating a snack or drinking a liquid rich in glucose. The diagnosis is based on a very low blood sugar (< 2 mmol/L) and a high level of insulin and C-peptide (indicative of endogenous insulin). The main differential diagnosis is self-administration of insulin.

Gastrinoma causes very high gastric acid secretion, resulting in refractory multiple peptic ulcers, often of a severe nature (Zollinger–Ellison syndrome), and sometimes diarrhea. There is commonly a history of gastric or duodenal perforation or hemorrhage, necessitating emergency surgery on one or more occasion. The diagnosis is based on finding high serum gastrin levels (> 1000 pg/mL, or > 200 pg/mL after secretin stimulation) in a patient who is not acholhydric and is producing acid. Gastrin levels may also be elevated by histamine H2-receptor blockers, proton-pump inhibitors or *Helicobacter pylori* infection, but are rarely above 400 pg/ml in these situations.

Glucagonoma causes a characteristic necrolytic migratory erythema of the skin, often starting in the groin and perineum, and may also affect the oral mucosa. Other features may include attacks of hyperglycemia, stomatitis, vulvitis, anemia, rash, weight loss, diarrhea and psychiatric disturbances. High plasma glucagon levels are invariably found.

Vasoactive intestinal polypeptide tumor. A VIPoma causes watery diarrhea and hypokalemia (Verner–Morrison syndrome). This results in massive intestinal loss of sodium and bicarbonate, leading to hypovolemia, hypokalemia and achlorhydria or metabolic acidosis. There may be impaired glucose tolerance (VIP causes mild insulin resistance) and hypercalcemia. The diagnosis is clinched by high plasma levels of VIP.

Carcinoid tumors only cause symptoms if there are large-volume hepatic metastases. They are distinct clinical, histological and biological tumors secreting serotonin, demonstrated by the presence of high levels of its derivative (5-hidroxy indol acetic acid) in urine.

Somatostatinoma and pancreatic polypeptide tumor do not cause distinct clinical syndromes and should be distinguished from non-functioning NETs.

Non-functioning pNETs are usually large when diagnosed, frequently with liver metastases. Consequently, the symptoms are non-specific and include abdominal pain, weight loss and jaundice.

Localization of tumors. High vascularity and the presence of somatostatin receptors characterize pNETs. Most gastrinomas, but only half of insulinomas, have somatostatin receptors. These features are important in localizing tumors, which can often be very small. Localization is straightforward in 90% of cases but can be very difficult in the remainder, requiring a range of investigations (Table 12.3), including contrast-enhanced multidetector CT, MRI (Figure 12.2), EUS (Figure 12.3) and somatostatin receptor scintigraphy.

TABLE 12.3

Investigations for localizing pancreatic neuroendocrine tumors

- Multidetector computed tomography
- Magnetic resonance imaging
- Somatostatin receptor scintigraphy (octreotide scan)
- Scintigraphy using radiolabeled meta-iodobenzylguanidine
- Endoscopic ultrasonography
- Intraoperative ultrasonography
- Selective pancreatic angiography
- Hepatic portal venous sampling and hormone assay

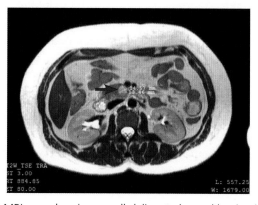

Figure 12.2 MRI scan showing a well-delineated round benign insulinoma in a young patient with hypoglycemic hyperinsulinemia.

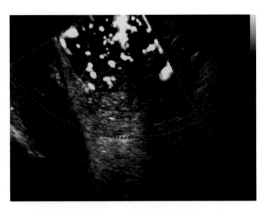

Figure 12.3 Contrast-enhanced power Doppler endoscopic ultrasound showing a hypervascular pancreatic neuroendocrine tumor localized at the level of the pancreatic head.

Imaging. Most pNETs are hypervascular on imaging, thus they are easily differentiated using contrast studies with transabdominal ultrasound, CT, MRI or angiography. Nevertheless, small tumors (insulinomas, gastrinomas, carcinoids) less than 10 mm in size are frequently missed by these imaging studies, being evident only on EUS combined with EUS-guided fine needle aspiration (FNA), which has an accuracy exceeding 90% for intrapancreatic NETs. EUS is also helpful for patients with MEN type-1 or VHL syndrome.

Somatostatin receptor scintigraphy is useful to localize various small pNETs, since they express somatostatin receptors which bind somatostatin analogs (octreotide, lanreotide). Radiolabeled somatostatin analogs such as [111In]-diethylenetriaminepentaacetic acid–octreotide are therefore used to localize pNETs (octreotide scanning). The method can be combined with CT or single photon emission computed tomography, which allows the detection of the primary tumor as well as liver metastases. Positron emission tomography, for example with [68]gallium-labeled somatostatin analogs, might be used more in the future.

Screening is usually based on MRI plus EUS and is indicated in patients with inherited pNETs (see page 138). It is used to identify pancreatic and extrapancreatic tumors in order to permit timely medical and surgical intervention.

Biopsy. The distinction between benign and malignant pNETs is difficult on histological grounds, but a high mitotic index is suggestive of malignancy. The risk of malignancy increases with tumor size (more than 2–3 cm). In principle, insulinomas tend to be benign, whereas all other pNETs have an increased propensity to malignancy.

A Ki-67 proliferative index may be performed in the biopsies of pNETs to assess aggressiveness, potential malignant behavior and to decide treatment.

Management. Patients with pNETs need to be managed by a multidisciplinary team that includes specialist endocrinologists, gastroenterologists, radiologists and pancreatic surgeons.

Medical treatment. The syndromes associated with all of these tumors, except for insulinoma, can be managed medically during the wait for surgery or, if there is metastatic disease, with a long-acting somatostatin receptor antagonist (octreotide long-acting release or lanreotide slow release). Although antitumor efficacy of somatostatin analogs is rather weak, there is disease stabilization in more than 50% of patients. Surgical tumor debulking is commonly undertaken, since the symptoms may still be difficult to control with somatostatin receptor antagonists.

Proton-pump inhibitors will effectively reduce gastric acid secretion from gastrinomas but will not prevent tumor growth and metastases.

Radionuclide therapy. Metastatic tumors that can be imaged by somatostatin receptor scintigraphy can be treated by radionuclide tagged to the somatostatin analog. An alternative is the use of radiolabeled meta-iodobenzylguanide (MIBG), a catecholamine analog. Active amine precursor uptake-1 mechanisms that can internalize MIBG are expressed by pNETs, resulting in the incorporation of MIBG into cytoplasmic neurosecretory granules.

Surgery. In general, pNETs have a good prognosis, provided complete resection of the primary tumor, lymph node and even hepatic metastases is undertaken. Most small insulinomas and gastrinomas are benign but cannot be managed well by medical measures and require removal. They can be resected by simple enucleation, while larger tumors can be subjected to more extensive pancreatic resections, for example Whipple pancreatoduodenectomy.

Radical resection is required for pNETs other than insulinomas as they tend to be malignant. Malignancy in insulinoma is indicated by the presence of lymph-node metastases, and a formal pancreatic resection is therefore also required. Gastrinomas are often multiple and are commonly found in the duodenal wall. Surgical resection is the only procedure that will provide a cure with a normal life expectancy.

Non-functioning pNETs have an unpredictable prognosis, even with surgical resection. However, surgical resection should be undertaken, when it is possible.

Chemotherapy. The response of pNETs to chemotherapy is disappointing. However, chemotherapy may be useful for patients with poorly differentiated NETs with a high proliferation index. Advanced pNETs may benefit from different chemotherapy regimens, including temozolomide- or streptozocine-based therapies. Newer agents are available, such as mTOR inhibitors (everolimus), alone or in combination with somatostatin analogs (octreotide long-acting release or lanreotide slow release). Other antiangiogenic drugs such as bevacizumab, sunitinib, sorafenib and pazopanib also have significant antitumor effects in pNETs.

Inherited pancreatic neuroendocrine tumors

There are four known syndromes and all are inherited in an autosomal-dominant manner. A patient with one of these syndromes requires genetic counseling and appropriate genetic testing.

Multiple endocrine neoplasia type-1 is caused by the *MEN1* gene and is characterized by tumors in the parathyroid and enteropancreatic endocrine tissues, and the anterior pituitary (mainly prolactinomas). The typical age at diagnosis is 20–40 years, and penetrance is nearly 100% at 50 years of age. Multiple facial angiofibromas occur in 85% of patients. The spectrum of pancreatic islet tumors comprises:

- gastrinomas in 25–67%
- insulinomas in 10–34%
- non-functioning tumors, including pancreatic polypeptide tumors (PPomas), in 10–50%
- glucagonomas in 3–8%
- vasoactive intestinal polypeptide tumors (VIPomas) in 1–5%
- somatostatinomas in less than 1%.

The major feature is diffuse microadenomatosis, with a tumor diameter ranging from 300 μm to 5 mm, usually associated with one or more larger tumors. Patients with MEN-1 type-1 are at increased risk of premature death at a median age of 46–48 years.

von Hippel–Lindau (VHL) syndrome is a rare disease caused by mutation in the *VHL* gene. Hypervascular neurological (central nervous hemangioblastomas and retinal angiomas), renal (clear cell carcinomas) and adrenal (pheochromocytomas) tumors are the commonly presenting lesions. Multiple pancreatic cysts are common and are invariably benign. In 12% of cases the pancreas may be the only organ affected.

The mean age at detection of pancreatic lesions is 38 years. Endolymphatic sac tumors and multiple pancreatic cysts, both of which are rare in the general population, suggest carrier status. The mean age at death without intervention is 41 years, with the most common cause of death being metastatic renal cell carcinoma or neurological complications from cerebellar hemangioblastomas.

Neurofibromatosis type 1 (NF-1) is a common inherited autosomal dominant disorder. It affects about 1 in 3000–4000 live births and is caused by the *NF-1* gene. In around 20% of patients the gastrointestinal tract is involved, with hyperplasia of submucosal or myenteric nerve plexuses, gastrointestinal stromal tumors, periampullary carcinoids, pheochromocytomas, periampullary paragangliomas, gastrointestinal adenocarcinomas and, rarely, pNETs, most frequently duodenal somatostatinomas.

Tuberous sclerosis (TSC) is a rare autosomal dominant genetic disorder resulting from mutation in the *TSC1* or *TSC2* genes. The major feature is the formation of hamartomas and neoplasms in multiple organs (brain, heart, kidney, skin) and, rarely, pNETs.

Other tumor types

Cystic pancreatic tumors. Cystic neoplasms need to be distinguished from pseudocysts secondary to acute or chronic pancreatitis. These tumors include serous cystadenomas, mucinous cystadenomas, mucinous cystadenocarcinomas, intraductal papillary mucinous neoplasms and other rare cystic lesions (cystic neuroendocrine tumors, etc.). Diagnosis is made by CT (Figure 12.4) or MRI with magnetic resonance cholangiopancreatography sequences (Figure 12.5), usually followed by EUS-guided FNA and analysis of the cystic fluid (Figure 12.6).

Serous cystadenomas are almost invariably benign, usually occur in women and are often left-sided. These tumors are harmless and may be observed serially using CT or EUS.

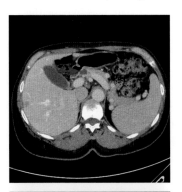

Figure 12.4 Contrast-enhanced CT image of a mucinous cystadenoma visualized at the level of the pancreatic head.

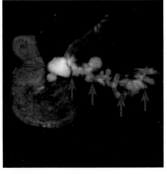

Figure 12.5 Magnetic resonance cholangiopancreatography image showing a dilated main pancreatic duct with multiple dilations of the side branches, indicating a typical mixed type intrapapillary mucinous neoplasm.

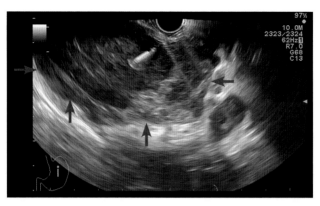

Figure 12.6 Endoscopic ultrasonography-guided fine needle aspiration in a mucinous tumor at the level of the liquid part of a mixed intraductal papillary mucinous neoplasm containing thick viscous mucin, which is difficult to extract by aspiration.

Mucinous cystadenomas and cystadenocarcinomas by definition contain mucin. Mucinous cystadenomas are premalignant and, along with cystadenocarcinomas, warrant radical excision.

Intraductal papillary mucinous neoplasms are being increasingly recognized. Pathognomonic features include an irregularly dilated main pancreatic duct containing thick mucus that is readily observed being extruded from the ampulla on endoscopy and/or one or more pancreatic cysts. The cysts develop either from the main pancreatic duct or from side branches. Intraductal papillary neoplasms with main pancreatic duct cysts are more likely to be malignant or progress to malignancy than neoplasms with side-branch cysts. Partial radical resection or total pancreatectomy is necessary in appropriate patients.

Multiple benign cysts may be a feature of polycystic kidney or renal syndrome, part of the VHL syndrome, or may indicate carrier status of the VHL gene.

Other malignant cystic lesions. A variety of pancreatic malignancies may contain cystic elements, including pancreatic ductal adenocarcinoma and neuroendocrine tumors.

Pancreatic lymphoma. By definition pancreatic lymphoma is restricted to the pancreas and draining lymph nodes. Resection should be undertaken where possible. If this is not feasible chemotherapy should be tried, although pancreatic lymphomas respond poorly.

Metastases to the pancreas. The pancreas is a site for the spread of metastases from cancers originating in the abdomen, breast, bronchus or skin (melanoma). Sometimes these metastases are isolated, in which case radical resection is the treatment of choice.

Future trends
- Improved preoperative classification to permit more accurate decision making regarding clinical management.
- Molecular profiling to enable accurate distinction between tumor types.
- Specific medical treatments for the different tumor types.
- Improved surveillance in patients with inherited pNETs.
- Better understanding of the malignant behavior of cystic pancreatic neoplasms based on molecular markers in cystic fluid.

Key points – unusual tumors of the pancreas and ampulla of Vater

- Tumor types that occur in the ampullary and periampullary regions may have a much better prognosis than pancreatic adenocarcinoma.
- Patients with pancreatic neuroendocrine tumors need to be managed by a multidisciplinary team.
- Neuroendocrine tumors should usually be removed surgically.
- Patients with inherited neuroendocrine tumors require genetic counseling and long-term follow-up for pancreatic and other tumor types.
- Cystic pancreatic tumors need to be differentiated from pancreatic pseudocysts, but only a minority need resection at the time of diagnosis.
- Solitary metastases to the pancreas may be worth resecting.

Key references

Al-Hawary MM, Kaza RK, Azar SF et al. Mimics of pancreatic ductal adenocarcinoma. *Cancer Imaging* 2013;13:342–9.

Bhutani MS, Gupta V, Guha S et al. Pancreatic cyst fluid analysis – a review. *J Gastrointestin Liver Dis* 2011;20:175–80.

El Hajj II, Coté GA. Endoscopic diagnosis and management of ampullary lesions. *Gastrointest Endosc Clin N Am* 2013;23:95–109.

Hatzaras I, George N, Muscarella P et al. Predictors of survival in periampullary cancers following pancreaticoduodenectomy. *Ann Surg Oncol* 2010;17:991–7.

Hutchins GF, Draganov PV. Cystic neoplasms of the pancreas: a diagnostic challenge. *World J Gastroenterol* 2009;15:48–54.

Ito T, Igarashi H, Jensen RT. Pancreatic neuroendocrine tumors: clinical features, diagnosis and medical treatment: advances. *Best Pract Res Clin Gastroenterol* 2012; 26:737–53.

Kim KW, Krajewski KM, Nishino M et al. Update on the management of gastroenteropancreatic neuroendocrine tumors with emphasis on the role of imaging. *AJR Am J Roentgenol* 2013;201:811–24.

Kulke MH, Anthony LB, Bushnell DL et al. NANETS treatment guidelines: well-differentiated neuroendocrine tumors of the stomach and pancreas. *Pancreas* 2010;39:735–52.

Kulke MH, Shah MH, Benson AB 3rd et al. Neuroendocrine tumors, version 1.2015. *J Natl Compr Canc Netw* 2015;13:78–108.

Matthaei H, Schulick RD, Hruban RH, Maitra A. Cystic precursors to invasive pancreatic cancer. *Nat Rev Gastroenterol Hepatol* 2011;8:141–50.

Öberg K, Knigge U, Kwekkeboom D et al. Neuroendocrine gastro-entero-pancreatic tumors: ESMO Clinical Practice Guidelines for diagnosis, treatment and follow-up. *Ann Oncol* 2012;23(Suppl 7):v124–30.

Perysinakis I, Margaris I, Kouraklis G. Ampullary cancer – a separate clinical entity? *Histopathology* 2014;64:759–68.

Puli SR, Kalva N, Bechtold ML et al. Diagnostic accuracy of endoscopic ultrasound in pancreatic neuroendocrine tumors: a systematic review and meta analysis. *World J Gastroenterol* 2013;19:3678–84.

Ramfidis VS, Syrigos KN, Saif MW. Ampullary and periampullary adenocarcinoma: new challenges in management of recurrence. *JOP* 2013;14:158–60.

Sahani DV, Kambadakone A, Macari M et al. Diagnosis and management of cystic pancreatic lesions. *AJR Am J Roentgenol* 2013;200:343–54.

Zbar AP, Maor Y, Czerniak A. Imaging tumours of the ampulla of Vater. *Surg Oncol* 2012;21:293–8.

Useful resources

UK
British Society of
Gastroenterology
Tel: +44 (0)20 7935 3150
www.bsg.org.uk

Pancreatic Cancer UK
Tel: +44 (0)20 3535 7090
www.pancreaticcancer.org.uk

USA
American Gastroenterological
Association
Tel: +1 301 654 2055
www.gastro.org

American Pancreatic Association
Tel: +1 305 243 6039
apa@miami.edu
www.american-pancreatic-
association.org

American Society for Clinical
Oncology (ASCO)
Tel: +1 571 483 1780
Toll-free: 888 651 3038
contactus@cancer.net
www.asco.org

National Cancer Institute
Tel: +1 800 422 6237
www.cancer.gov/cancertopics/types/
pancreatic

National Pancreas Foundation
Tel: +1 301 961 1508
Toll free: 866 726 2737
info@pancreasfoundation.org
www.pancreasfoundation.org

Pancreas Cancer Web
Johns Hopkins University
www.path.jhu.edu/pancreas

Pancreas.org
www.pancreas.org

Pancreatica
Tel: +1 831 658 0600
info@pancreatica.org
www.pancreatica.org

Pancreatic Cancer Action
Network (PanCAN)
Tel: +1 310 725 0025
Toll free: 877 573 9971
info@pancan.org
www.pancan.org

Society of Gastroenterology
Nurses and Associates
Tel: 800 245 7462
info@sgna.org
www.sgna.org

International

Australasian Pancreatic Club
Tel: +61 2 4348 4680
info@pancreas.org.au
www.pancreas.org.au

European Society of
Gastroenterology and Endoscopy
Nurses and Associates
Tel: +49 8459 323941
www.esgena.org

European Society of
Gastrointestinal Endoscopy
Tel: +49 89 907 7936-11
www.esge.com

International Association of
Pancreatology
Tel: +91 11 2659 4425
www.internationalpancreatology.
org

Pancare Foundation (Australia)
Tel: 1300 881 698
info@pancare.org.au
www.pancare.org.au

Pancreatic Cancer Canada
Tel: 1 888 726 2269
info@pancancanada.ca
www.pancreaticcancercanada.ca

World Endoscopy Organization
Tel: +49 89 907 7936-12
secretariat@worldendo.org
www.worldendo.org

Index

FastTest

**You've read the book ... now test yourself
with key questions from the authors**

- Go to the FastTest for this title
  FREE at fastfacts.com

- Approximate time **10 minutes**

- For best retention of the key issues, try taking the
  FastTest before and after reading

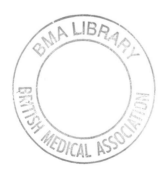

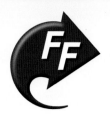
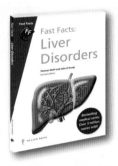
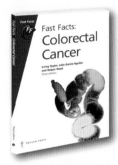
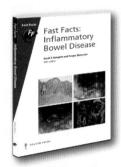
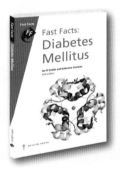
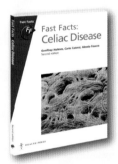
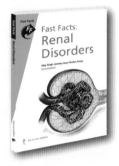
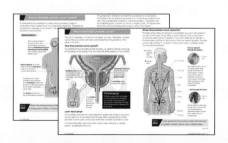

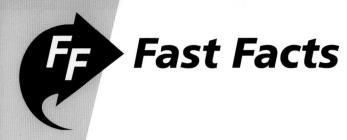

Fast Facts

Reading for results
(and tests worth taking)

With so much to read these days, you need to be selective ...

Was this Fast Facts well worth reading?

Has it helped you make good health decisions?

Did it trigger new ideas you'd like to explore?

If so, please post them in the comments box on the relevant page on **www.fastfacts.com**, and check out fellow readers' insights while you're there.

This is also the place to leave questions for the authors' consideration, and to spend 10 minutes on the free **FastTest** to ensure those key points really sunk in, and that you are set to apply them – **result!**

This Fast Facts has helped me make good health decisions:

| ✔ | YES |
| ✘ | NO | | SUBMIT | ❯ |

27
Good health decisions

Comments for the authors

Name:

Comment:

Country: Please select ▾

ADD COMMENT ❯

---

fastfacts.com